FACING CANCER WITH AN ATTITUDE

BEYOND SURVIVORSHIP

Health

Dear Marcia,

May you keep managing the Life Force within with skillful means towards Well Being with Lovingkindness

Kindly,
Pierre

To Selma, the loving partner in this life, both of us leading people towards wellbeing.

May my children, Heidi, Claire and Asha continue to thrive with their loved ones.

Acknowledgments

I am grateful for all the superb teachers and mentors in my life who inspired, assisted and surprised me with their profound skills to align body, mind, heart and spirit, allowing the move from drifting to shifting views about the self and the places I inhabited throughout the years to the present moment.

I am grateful for John McCann, MD, who was my oncologist, two decades ago, a true mensch!

There are not enough pages to mention all the names. I give credit to a few teachers from the spiritual realms, their feet well grounded in day to day living among us:

Roshi Joan Halifax, Chokyi Nyima, S. N Goenka, Sogyal Rinpoche, Pema Chodron, His Holiness the Dalai Lama, Tsoknyi Rinpoche, Ayya Khema, Allan Wallace, Sharon Salzberg, Matthieu Ricard and many more.

In the field of neurobiology, psychiatry, psychology, medicine, most of them also meditation practitioners:

Daniel Siegel MD, Rachel Naomi Remen MD, Daniel Goleman PhD, John Welwood PhD, Jon Kabat Zinn PhD, Gabor Mate, MD.

In the field of organizational management, I particularly appreciate the work of Peter Senge and Peter Block.

There are many others who had influence in my life, maybe not famous, whose name will not be available, yet deserve praise for listening, their support and bearing witness to the many trials, aspirations and changes in my life.

I am grateful for two polished editors, that put up with my requests, asking many questions and giving sound advice while my patience wasn't always front and center in my interactions with them. Mary Hanson, guided me during the first two years in the midst of Covid, sorting ideas out of a maze of mangled words and many concepts during the first draft.

Ayshea Wild assisted me in rewriting the book a second time as I decided to use the word "attitude" as chapter titles, sorting out pieces of writing from existing chapters and writing new ones. She always ended her emails with " gentle" after requesting changes, putting out new ideas or checking in about new content that needed to be reconsidered and rewritten by me. She used very kind measures and offered many ideas, being a great coach for a frustrated novice writer. I owe both of them much gratitude for their attention to details and their suggestions in differentiating the trees from the forest…

I want to honor the cancer patients, whose journey I brought to life, whose fictitious names are mentioned in the book to illustrate and support ideas and beliefs that I put forth about living beyond survivorship.

I also want to give credit to Zach Andrew, senior publisher manager from Amazon Publishing Solutions, for formatting and editing the text, designing the cover and giving the book the final attention it needed.

Table of Contents

"Much good can come from an open mind engagement with the process that disease represents.

It may not be the guest we ever desire, but a modicum of hospitality, welcoming the unwelcome, so to speak costs nothing.

It might even lead to an opportunity to find out why this particular visitor has come to call, and what it might tell us about our lives."

Gabor Mate

The Myth of Normal

Introduction

When you receive a cancer diagnosis, the ground vanishes from under your feet. You feel like you are hanging from a branch by your teeth, more than fifty feet from terra firma, where someone below asks: "What is the meaning and purpose of your life?" If you respond, you will surely plummet to the ground. If you don't respond, the result won't be any better.

After the initial shock, and accompanying constriction of the mind and body, an inner accounting is necessary. This involves adopting a mindset that envisions well-being, regardless of the outcome of the disease. As I have experienced personally, and witnessed in others, when we meet our edges and work with them, vivid purpose and meaning emerge, opening the door for transformation to take place.

People who have been diagnosed with cancer and come out of their struggle alive after a lengthy cancer journey often call themselves "survivors." This designation is fundamentally inadequate, because survivorship connotes meeting basic needs and winning battles. It is possible, however, for the journey to culminate in well-being, thriving, and self-actualization.

Well-being is not just about being cancer-free. It is about valuing life from a whole new perspective, living with the understanding that every moment is fresh, believing that every breath honors life with energy and clarity. In a state of well-being, we are open to expanding the heart and mind, becoming larger than any problem we encounter, overcoming adversity, and finding a higher purpose. We have the power within us to live more fully than we have in the past and to bring out the basic goodness in ourselves and others.

My experiences with allopathic and holistic treatments lead me to believe that both are essential in the process of recovery. For so long, curing cancer has been fundamentally relegated to the work of clinicians and researchers, while healing has been the primary responsibility and task of the patient. We need to reassess this division. Wherever you are on your journey, improving your quality of life here and now is invaluable, whatever the future holds.

Beyond Survivorship is not a manual for dying; it is a framework for reconnecting with our physical, emotional, and mind states. There are infinite opportunities to make our minds serviceable to ourselves, meet our innate goodness, and acknowledge new possibilities. This book will show you how to adjust your mindset and gain equanimity, rather than capitulate and drown in a sea of limitations and despair. It offers a comprehensive plan to broaden your view by focusing on the connection between body and mind. The cancer journey doesn't need to be a war against a foreign entity in your body. Instead, it can offer new ways for you to open up to the mysteries that life has to offer.

In times of crisis, we discover ways to transform ourselves. In Western culture we see crisis as an unwanted, annoying burden that often brings with it long-term obstacles and consequences. The Chinese symbol for crisis has, instead, two interesting specific meanings: danger and opportunity. All of us face unfavorable experiences in life that we consider dangerous. The opportunity for preserving or reclaiming our well-being compels us to learn lessons and integrate them into our lives. Overall wellness entails matters of the heart, mind, and spirit, as well as the body. The mind is most important; without it, we cannot be aware of anything.

In December 2001, I was diagnosed with a stage IV transitional cell carcinoma and given a timeline of four-to-six months before fatal cancer cells were supposed to overtake my being. As much as I wanted to have a sense of what the future held, I rejected this sudden deadline, which was solely based on scientific data and, in my opinion, only looked at the danger. I didn't settle for becoming a statistic. The prognosis gave me some time to attempt to redirect the stubborn, destructive trajectory of the cancer cells. I used my defiance not just to survive, but to come out on the other side free of both cancer and my habitual, limiting patterns. I gained new purpose, meaning, and understanding, as well as more time.

For the past seventeen years, I have been offering support groups, individual sessions, and mindfulness practices to people who have been diagnosed with cancer. These rewarding experiences have filled me with humility and grace. Through my engagement with patients, I have learned to discern what brings them vitality and resilience, and the difference between those who are able to find peace in the midst of their illness and those who have not attained even a glimmer of serenity. Every person who has or has had cancer remembers the exact date they received their diagnosis. BC (Before Cancer) is the new marker of time. Even chemo brains never forget that date. I have seen the moment of cancer diagnosis open up a connection to the soul and also cause a temporary descent into a deep well of grief for a lost way of life.

Over time, I have observed certain traits that support patients and caregivers on the journey toward physical, emotional, and spiritual health. Those who focus on living fully in the moment, connecting with community, and committing to a less self-absorbed perspective fare better than those who choose isolation. No matter how feeble the life force might reveal itself to be during illness, patients who engage with caregivers and other patients with similar needs manage to open up, release pent-up emotions, and find a path that leads them home to themselves again and again.

People who make beneficial changes adopt an enduring attitude that goes beyond coping. I feel compelled to share the choices and skills sets needed to go through the process of self-transformation. This multi-level guide advocates for adopting an attitude that harnesses awareness and introspection, through different mind and heart states, to change neural pathways in the brain and promote comprehensive health.

Part One of the book tells the story of my own cancer journey. Part Two uses the acronym ATTITUDE, which stands for assault, terror, trauma, intervention, toll, understanding, dependence, and equanimity, to define the stages of a transformative approach to cancer, a different kind of journey. One definition, from BusinessDictionary.com, says attitude is the "predisposition or tendency to respond toward an idea or situation, it influences our choice of action and responses to stimuli and challenges." Bruce Lipton, in *The Biology of Belief,* writes that in changing our lifestyle, beliefs, and perceptions, we change our genetic expression. How we interpret our world is translated by the brain into chemical information that adjusts our behavior and interpretations. This allows our genes to manifest either in a functional or dysfunctional state of health. We can limit or expand our choices with our attitude. Changing it requires both forward momentum and stepping back to discern what is needed from moment to moment.

This book is intended as a resource for cancer patients, caregivers, chaplains, and clinicians working in oncology, palliative care, and hospice. The book draws on personal experience, mindfulness practices, Buddhist teachings and psychology, neurobiology, case studies of cancer patients, and the field of epigenetics. The meditations within the chapters are meant to calm the mind and open the heart, and the exercises are for putting ideas into direct practice, bringing understanding about the nature and depth of our common humanity and how to engage with it.

The initial stage of the journey occurs pre-diagnosis. This is the assault on the body by rogue cells. Bouts can last several years from inception to remission or death. We do not know for sure what gives malignant cells the impetus to propagate and invade tissue and organs. We do know that chronic stress and cortisol exposure decrease telomere supplies, which make cells die or become pro-inflammatory with certain mutations, which makes some people more likely to develop cancer (NCBI). Any invasion of the body by dangerous, rogue cells, causes us to reconsider how we live our lives and what measures to pursue to actualize change.

With diagnosis, terror arises. We experience fear, despair, and helplessness, while obsessing and indulging in catastrophic thinking. It is not uncommon to experience shock and become temporarily immobilized with the news, regardless of the severity of the diagnosis. All the attention is on specific dysfunctional body parts, at the expense of the whole being and it's emotional, cognitive, and spiritual considerations.

Trauma ensues from dealing with the unknown, being subjected to chemotherapy, and experiencing loneliness. We must muster enough courage, stamina, and discernment to concentrate on interrupting the trajectory of rogue cells in the body, by integrating new mind and heart-element practices with the support of medical interventions.

As we face our mortality, introspective, sober intervention becomes necessary. We explore strategies, evaluating what might do more harm than good, letting go of unbeneficial habits. Efforts to build on positive, lasting traits begin to guide us toward well-being.

We acknowledge the extensive physical, emotional, and cognitive toll of the journey. We explore and gather new resources and skills. There is a lot to take care of when, paradoxically, our energy is waning. We accept the challenge to envision a healthy life, wholeheartedly committing to make the rogue cells vanish, or prevent their resurgence before or after remission.

Understanding there is potential for posttraumatic growth, we adopt a new vision. This is a long journey of re-orientation and re-evaluation. We release habitual constructs that no longer serve us. We drop deep into our interior vistas to truly see and redefine ourselves. Then we can regulate overwhelming emotions, create balance between doing and being, and reconnect to the world around us better. We are like fishermen in a tsunami, eschewing retreat and sailing toward the vast sea to avoid the overwhelming force of the treacherous underlying currents. We face our fears, acknowledging we have limited control over our lives.

Dependence on our own capacity to heal, and find peace and comfort, makes it possible for us to bond with others as they join us on the journey. We need healthy food, physical activity, sound values, a sane ethical outlook, and the sense of connection that therapy and support groups provide. Being part of a community of vital and constructive members helps us to regain some cohesion. We cultivate clarity and kindness as we gain ample insights from the hardship we experience. We don't just put food and medicine in our bodies; we also take in dizzying amounts of information. Unless we are able to integrate this information and deconstruct the assumptions, beliefs, and ideas that have influenced and overpowered us, the "dis-ease" can worsen. Integration leads to self-efficacy, which allows us to proceed with a strong feeling of confidence.

Equanimity can be found by redefining one's sense of meaning and purpose, living fully in the present, and eventually flourishing. Our mindset, or attitude, during illness, personal conflicts, and other tribulations has either beneficial or adverse consequences, depending on whether we stand firmly in the central axis of our being. This is a place within us that is like a firmly rooted willow tree under the pressure of strong winds. It bends and then resumes its natural stance once the force of the wind subsides, demonstrating tremendous resilience. This is the place of compassion: the wish to alleviate suffering and its causes. Compassion is cultivated through the practice of loving-kindness. Now we accept ourselves with all our assets and liabilities, letting go of judgment, honoring discernment, and determining what is uplifting and what is harmful.

ATTITUDE establishes a new foundation with which to support wholesome choices and pursue a new lease on life. Personal growth, despite all the problems of our lives, never needs to stop. Following your mind and heart will give you a sense of direction that validates your unique potential, sound strategies, and noble values. I hope this book serves you well. Never give up. Give it your all. Claim your innate gift of being fully alive.

Some of the materials and meditations have been drawn from different cultures and oral transmissions from time immemorial. Many of the exercises, concepts are personal interpretations from them and I honor all the teachings that have been passed on and brought to my attention in many different settings and platforms. I am blessed to have been exposed to them over the past forty five years or so and integrate them in my life, on an ongoing basis.

The Invitation

It doesn't interest me
what you do for a living.
I want to know
what you ache for
and if you dare to dream
of meeting your heart's longing.

It doesn't interest me
how old you are.
I want to know
if you will risk
looking like a fool
for love
for your dream
for the adventure of being alive.

It doesn't interest me
what planets are
squaring your moon...
I want to know
if you have touched
the center of your own sorrow
if you have been opened
by life's betrayals
or have become shriveled and closed
from fear of further pain.

I want to know
if you can sit with pain
mine or your own
without moving to hide it
or fade it
or fix it.

I want to know

if you can be with joy
mine or your own
if you can dance with wildness
and let the ecstasy fill you
to the tips of your fingers and toes
without cautioning us
to be careful
to be realistic
to remember the limitations
of being human.

It doesn't interest me
if the story you are telling me
is true.
I want to know if you can
disappoint another
to be true to yourself.
If you can bear
the accusation of betrayal
and not betray your own soul.
If you can be faithless
and therefore trustworthy.

I want to know if you can see Beauty
even when it's not pretty
every day.
And if you can source your own life
from its presence.

I want to know
if you can live with failure
yours and mine
and still stand at the edge of the lake
and shout to the silver of the full moon,
"Yes."

It doesn't interest me
to know where you live
or how much money you have.

I want to know if you can get up
after the night of grief and despair

weary and bruised to the bone
and do what needs to be done
to feed the children.

It doesn't interest me
who you know
or how you came to be here.
I want to know if you will stand
in the center of the fire
with me
and not shrink back.

It doesn't interest me
where or what or with whom
you have studied.
I want to know
what sustains you
from the inside
when all else falls away.

I want to know
if you can be alone
with yourself
and if you truly like
the company you keep
in the empty moments.

(by Oriah Mountain Dreamer 1999)

PART ONE:
MY STORY

I was born in Alsace, France, an area bordering Germany and Switzerland. I was brought up in a cul-de-sac, in a small village surrounded by mountains, with a population of no more than nine hundred. It looked like a scene from Heidi. There were few distractions; our family had no TV. We did not even have a refrigerator until I was about ten years old. We were more fortunate than neighboring families, because my dad was the only person holding a white-collar job following the Second World War in an area of struggling factories, small individual farms, and private vineyards.

I was eventually joined by two younger sisters. We took walks, skied, and luged in the winter, and in summer we biked and hiked, picking fruit from the many private orchards and vineyards lodged on the steep slopes of the surrounding southern hills. On Sundays after Mass, we played games outside, while the men went to the local restaurant for an aperitif and the women fixed lunch. It was a quiet area, and the pace was slow and balanced. People would get up early and go to bed after dusk. They had large family gatherings around food on the weekends. The food was all natural, seasonal, and not as varied as what we have today. Tropical fruits, such as dates, figs, and oranges, were a real treat and available only during winter holidays.

In those days, pollution was far less of a concern and few planes crossed the vast expanse of the sky. My father rode a motorcycle and was the first person in the village to own a car. He worked long hours as a contract lawyer, always serving people above and beyond the call of duty, which would upset my mother because dinner was often cold by the time he got home. His real passion was beekeeping. We loved to harvest white pine and chestnut honeys together, both of which had a deep, dark color. Often, after a rainy summer weekend day, my dad and I would compete in hunting for mushrooms, making sure we didn't run into wild boars. We collected wild blueberries, raspberries, strawberries, and quinces, which my mother and grandmother would use to make jams and pies. Many indigenous fruits were used to make a strong, tasty, widely cherished schnapps called eau-de-vie, or water of life. It had a very high alcohol content, and was used for drinking, mixing into baked goods, and treating colds and various other bodily ailments.

My father, my sisters, and I were dismissive of Mother's old-fashioned remedies and approach to wellness and preventive care. She would send her new slippers to the Vatican to be blessed before wearing them; we thought that was going a step too far. On the other hand, I am grateful that she introduced me to many healing herbs used for tea, and cooking, or as remedies for colds and other illnesses. Women would learn, and rely on, the benefits of the restorative properties of local plants, because there were no doctors in our village or surrounding area.

Mom used to make nettle soup for dinner, which energized us, our faces flushing from the high mineral content. Now I find it intriguing that one of my teachers in Tibet spent years in a cave mostly eating nettle soup offered him by villagers. But back then we didn't know that nettles were the main ingredient of the soup, until I followed her one day and discovered where the magic herb grew in abundance. Finding out that her soup was made of stinging nettles was reason never to eat it again. For us kids, the purpose of stinging nettles was for punishing our friends, knowing well the sharp pain from the plant would last for a while. The trick was to pick them by grasping them underneath the stems and leaves, moving the hand upward without getting stung. The little secret didn't last long; when word got out, we got reciprocal scourging.

When I was about nine years old, my mother asked me to see a man who was an intuitive healer with no conventional credentials. He told my mother that my left kidney wasn't functional at all. I don't recall if there was a treatment plan to remedy the condition. For a kid, a kidney has no relevance compared to a bike, a sled, roller skates, or skis. Through my early adult life this experience was largely forgotten, until the day of my cancer diagnosis.

At age ten I went to a private catholic boarding school led by Jesuits and Brothers of Joseph. The education was acceptable, but the dissonance between what was taught about religion and exhibited in the behavior of those wearing black robes was abhorrent. After a few years, I transferred to a more academic boarding school and then went to the university in Besançon, majoring in German language, literature, and philosophy. I was greatly influenced by Herman Hesse, Carl Jung, Rainer Maria Rilke, Goethe, and other writers who had an interest in eastern religions, psychology, spirituality, and philosophy. I never graduated, because in 1968 the universities closed due to the political upheaval. Instead, I joined demonstrations against the government, the police force, and the army, overturning and burning cars and blocking streets. This was a great outlet for the rage I'd carried for a long time against people in uniform.

While teaching high school geography and German, I met an American woman who was struggling with the French language. We talked a lot after school and became fond of each other. Her visa was going to end, and she invited me to come to the United States. My father disapproved, so I waited until I was twenty-one and got my own passport. My parents and I said our goodbyes in Cannes. They couldn't believe that I was leaving, and I saw my father cry for the first time.

Nothing was going to change my mind. I'd wanted to leave Alsace from an early age because of all the trauma there from World War II. During weddings people would have fun the first day, then the second day not so much, and by the third day people were fighting. There were many unresolved issues right below the surface that would burst into the open after alcohol was consumed: memories about those who had resisted fighting and resentment about the women in the village who had married German soldiers. I wasn't interested in staying long; my plan was to go to China to learn Mandarin. But I got married and had children, my wife was hospitalized for several months, I took charge of the children and work, and I never left. Later, I went to college and received a BA in Psychology and Eastern Philosophy. A few years later I earned an MS in Organizational Management and Development, while raising three children.

During this period, I became interested in Buddhism. I loved the fact that the Buddha said to check out the teachings, not follow them blindly, and to draw your own conclusions from your experiences. When I lived in New York City, I was introduced to Sogyal Rinpoche, an inspiring teacher who wrote *The Tibetan Book of Living and Dying* and was involved, in England and other countries, with hospices and end-of-life care. He had a great sense of humor, deep insight, and a wonderful belly laugh. I attended his lectures and retreats and consequently met many more teachers. I also worked diligently and successfully for a single company through many take-overs. Because I never abdicated my two months of vacation each year, I balanced my life with my interest in Buddhist trainings all over the US and spent a month in Cannes as well.

Most of my work history consists of a variety of positions in the field of corporate healthcare in the U S and Canada. I was quite successful at developing programs, assessing market changes, setting up strategies to stay ahead of the competition, and gaining a differential edge for the companies I represented. After decades, and long hours in systems that seemed broken on so many levels, I grew tired of dealing with continuous and recurring problems. It felt like putting Band-Aids on ruptured arteries. By the time one crisis was fixed, another one had reared its ugly head. During this time, I traveled frequently for about twelve years, racking up miles on planes and cars throughout North America.

I continued my career in healthcare for many years out of fear that I would not to be able to support myself and my family if I quit. I changed companies a couple of times and navigated my way through corporate buyouts. At one point I wished to become sick just so I could stop running on what felt like a nonstop Machiavellian treadmill. Well, that desperate longing—born of losing heart and feeling stuck—was realized. I started experiencing a recurring pain in my lower-left front and back quadrant. I was brought up in a culture where one never complains or makes a fuss about physical pain short of becoming nonambulatory. I finally set up an appointment with a physician who gave me a diagnosis of "eating too fast," which was true but struck me as a bizarre conclusion. I felt relief, however, living with the illusion that my acute pain would go away on its own; the fear of discovering an actual malady was a much more dreadful possibility.

One night, I discharged blood in my urine. I still wasn't planning to ask for help, although I knew deep inside that this was a serious problem. My partner at the time noticed the discharge in the toilet, which I had declined to flush so as not to wake her during the night. She immediately took me to see my primary care physician, who recommended a urologist.

Meanwhile, I contacted a medical intuitive located in Maine, a physician still practicing and leading workshops to this day. The only information she had was my first name, phone number, and age. She shared with me what she was perceiving, moving from head to toe, describing energy levels and emotions in different parts of my body. When she came to my back, she disclosed, "Your left back quadrant is on fire, bright red. Your left kidney isn't functioning at all. It is as if a woman kicked you hard in that area. I think some big betrayal happened, not too long ago. She might have been involved with someone else you didn't know about. She treated you harshly when you figured it out. The other man gave her an emerald ring." I was stunned that she picked up so much accurate information, given the limited knowledge I had given her about myself.

In fact, I had worked closely with a married woman in the recent past. I was single at the time. We were fond of each other and became lovers. I broke one of my most important values: do not get involved with a married woman, because it never fails to create tremendous suffering, whether the people affected know about it consciously or not. I certainly did not wish to be in a relationship with a partner who was having an affair, though I did experience it a couple of times. I was surprised that I was so proficient at keeping this secret from my work colleagues. I eventually lost my job when I posed a challenge to a man positioned higher up in the company with whom she was having another extramarital affair.

The consultation with the medical intuitive suggested the emotional anguish and stress I had dealt with after my botched romance could be linked to the onset and exacerbation of my physical pain. I asked her if I was going to die. She replied, "I cannot answer that question. What

I would recommend is that you see your primary care physician immediately and make an appointment with a urologist to get several tests done. They will determine what the problem is and get you the services you need." I detected a sense of urgency for an immediate intervention. I thanked her, and the next day I followed up with my doctor.

After a few tests, I was told I had a tumor the size of a tennis ball that had broken through my left kidney, and the cancer had spread into the ureter. The urologist asked me to sign a contract pledging I would immediately contact another physician in Massachusetts, where I had planned to resettle. He was concerned about his liability around my condition and wasn't sure he could trust me to do something about it. I realized then that this was a critical and urgent problem, and that I was turning a new corner in my life. I was suddenly embarking on an unexpected journey down a winding, swollen river, on a small raft, in the dark of the night.

"Transitional carcinoma," were the resounding words from the oncologist. At first, I thought "transitional" meant temporary, as in moving on rapidly. It did not. It was an aggressive cancer whose pathway usually moves from the kidney into the bladder and goes up the other side to invade the remaining kidney. I've never heard of anyone surviving the cancer's trajectory beyond the bladder. I was given a stage IV diagnosis and a four-to-six-month survival prognosis. "You might want to get your things in order," was the ominous recommendation. It felt like someone had stuck a knife in my throat; I couldn't utter any words. An unusual and rare cancer— if I had ever wanted to be special, I could certainly consider myself so now.

The words "transitional carcinoma" kept resonating in my ears over and over, while the world suddenly turned upside-down. I became immobilized for a couple of weeks. No more terra firma! How could that be? I had spent a fortune in health food stores during my adult life and exercised fairly regularly. But the past was irrelevant, time was of the essence, and surgery was scheduled immediately, before I had the chance to relocate. The surgeon was kind and compassionate. I trusted him and his skills. My left kidney was excised and disposed of in a medical dump. He suggested I seek a second opinion from a urologist for further treatment.

After surgery, I waited five months before I had enough strength to undergo an aggressive chemo regimen. Before starting this invasive therapy, I joined a men's support group and saw an acupuncturist, who treated me with Chinese herbs and supplements, against the recommendation of my allopathic physicians. They worry, of course, that unconventional remedies contraindicate allopathic therapies. I figured I had nothing to lose! I will never know for sure what worked, but my hunch is that my never-give-up attitude influenced the elimination of rogue cells. BC, I had always said that I would attempt suicide by slamming my car into a wall if I was afflicted with a terminal disease. However, I never considered the prospect once I received my diagnosis. We never know for sure how we will react in drastic times.

My oncologist put together a cocktail of five chemotherapeutic fluids with complicated names. Many patients become experts at reciting the names of their therapeutic drugs. I had no interest in remembering what they were called. I haven't forgotten their colors, though: red, blue, and yellow. There was very little evidence for what was working for this rare type of cancer, and no clinical trials were available twenty years ago. More was better! A strong mélange was in order.

I wasn't sure I wanted to go that route. I decided to participate in a ten-day silent retreat for executives, at an old inn situated in the Berkshires, with S. N. Goenka, a world-renowned meditation teacher from Burma, now called Myanmar. It wasn't the first ten-day retreat that I'd experienced, but this one was more meaningful than past retreats. I was in a large room with about 150 other corporate businesspeople, from all over the planet, sitting on cushions from 5 a.m. to 10 p.m. I was sitting in a chair, a privilege of being ill. My goals were to regain a calmer state of mind and eventually decide whether to undergo chemo or not. During the retreat, I elected to go with the traditional treatment route. Whether it would work or not was important to me, but even more pressing was the fact that I knew my children were in favor of some kind of medical intervention, even though they'd never expressed a specific request.

The day my youngest daughter took me for my second round of chemo, I noticed fuzzy stuff flying around inside her car, the open windows letting in the hot summer air. It looked like dandelion seedpods spinning around in slow motion. It took me a while to realize that it was my own hair whirling around, falling off my head. Once I did, my stomach twisted into knots; I was familiar with cancer treatment side effects, but neither my body nor my mind were prepared for this sudden experience of evident loss! The whole world was revolving erratically— the hair, my mind, words, beliefs, everything was unhinged! My daughter quietly asked me if I wanted to have it cut when we arrived home. I didn't have an answer right away. I was lost in pregnant moments of silence.

My daughter's friend shaved my head that evening. My sons-in-law were happy that I had no hair; a shiny head just like them. These joking baldheads were trying to make light of the situation. I told them that if I didn't die, I would let my hair grow long again and I would have the last laugh. What they didn't know was that a few days later I lost my pubic, ear, and nose hair, and finally my eyebrows, in that order. My first granddaughter was two years old and was uncomfortable with my illness and new look. She didn't want to spend time with me. I looked like an alien, with a big head, no hair or eyebrows, and slightly leathery, yellow chemo-skin! Back then, looking helplessly different and with naked awareness, I had to laugh at the small ironies of life. I remember feeling the breeze on my bare head, which was so refreshing during those hot summer chemo-months; one unexpected benefit among many unpleasant side effects.

Shortly after, I attended a two-day retreat in Western Massachusetts taught by Tibetan lama Chökyi Nyima Rinpoche. Well-known psychologist Daniel Goleman, a neighbor of sorts, who had invited the lama for this retreat, didn't recognize me at first. I had attended a few workshops with him and his wife prior to the event. When I got him up to speed about my new predicament, he suggested I request a special healing from Rinpoche. I approached Rinpoche and asked him for a blessing. He inquired, "Which order of monks do you belong to?" "I am from the order of chemotherapy," I replied. Perhaps owing to a language barrier, he did not seem to understand that I was speaking in jest. His translator, Eric, explained my situation and gave him more specific information. Without a moment of hesitancy, the lama took my head in his hands and, with a serious look on his face, connected our foreheads together and prayed in Tibetan, suspended in time. Then he told me without hesitation, "You are going to be fine. Not to worry, I will have all the monks and nuns in Kathmandu pray for you for a full month." Initially, the strictly rational, familiar critic in my mind attempted to respond, "Yeah right," but my whole being had experienced a spacious heart-to-heart opening and absorbed the news from Rinpoche peacefully. I thanked him and took refuge in the dharma teachings. I was given a lineage name, Kunzang Sherab, which translates as "Vivid, Clear Knowledge."

This propitious meeting gave me confidence, strengthened my attitude, and reinforced my wish to start rerouting the rogue cells. While I was under the influence of chemo juices, I meditated and imagined honey and royal jelly flowing down my port. However, this image never lasted long, as I was besieged by worries about these unnatural-looking liquids dripping down my port and into my body, which didn't seem to be my real body. The weekly schedule for chemo was arduous: day one required three to four hours of treatment, day two a couple of hours, and on day three my sole kidney was flushed for an hour, all to be repeated for the remaining three weeks of the month. I never received the fourth week's colorful concoction because my white blood cell count was too low, and I was very nauseated, gagging and heaving, but unable to vomit. I've been drunk enough once in my life to experience the world spinning around while unable to empty my stomach. And another time, too, on a fishing boat, in seven-foot swells. I promised the strange gods of the ocean that I would do anything to be able to purge my queasiness or pass out, so I wouldn't keep seeing the waves slamming against the bathroom window. I finally did faint. When I regained consciousness, I declared I would never step on a fishing boat ever again. I have kept my promise to this day.

For the second month of chemo, I was required to give myself an injection, into any muscle, to boost my level of white blood cells. I gave that up after a couple of times; I hate needles and I envisioned my body being slowly rearranged like a complex puzzle, while my mind, blank, was nowhere to be found. I was willing to take a chance and skipped those shots. Instead, I juiced watermelon with the rind daily and took long Epsom salt baths at the recommendation of a friend I trusted fully. It was one of the hottest summers I can recall, and the watermelon did magic to my overheated chemo- and steroid-packed body.

After five months of colorful poison seeping into my body and excruciating physical and emotional distress, I became more and more exhausted. I felt like I was living in a swamp, motionless as an alligator, barely able to keep my eyes above the slime. I had no energy, just stared into blank space in pure mindlessness. Crawling from the futon to the bathroom and back seemed to take forever, but pleasantly reduced the boredom of staring at the small details on the ceiling, the lapis Medicine Buddha painting on the wall, or the clouds through the window. At night, awake for hours, I listened to the owls conversing from one hill to another, as well as occasional coyotes, yapping and lamenting under the blanket of the dark, endless, lingering nights. I just lay there, my thumbs interlocked over my beating heart, the rest of my body otherwise static. Five months later, I mobilized my body's energy to become more resilient, determined to keep breathing, and eventually regained stamina.

It is interesting to notice the predominant language of war in business management, politics, and illness, in which we fight for the sake of winning, struggle just to survive, and issue arbitrary or premature declarations of victory or articles of surrender. It struck me as odd to battle the cells in my own body, instead of redirecting them to die off. I questioned if, rather than allowing the cells to monopolize my body, I could possibly alter the trajectory of my internal functioning by shifting my mindset. Anything that is alive is moving and constantly changing. Looking back,

I consider this contemplation to have been an initial step in my attempt to understand how I might communicate consciously with the workings of my physiology. The speculation gave me an impetus to figure out how to relate to the disease. The diagnosis wasn't a terminal destination or fait accompli. There was still room to prevent the rogue cells from inflicting more chaos and taking over. I could improve the quality of my existence by reexamining my attitude toward life and death in general.

"I am not going to give up" became my motto, even though it required effort just to lie down, follow my breath, and hold on to my tender heart. I often felt at peace, grounded in being, coming home to myself. There was still a lot to live for, and my twenty years of meditation practice was a saving grace, allowing traits like equanimity, patience, and faith to surface in the midst of this uninvited drama. I realized how little control I had, and yet I saw unlimited opportunities to welcome everything that presented itself in my life. After a few months, the chemicals in my body slowly receded, along with a few remaining minor side effects. By using mindsight, which according to Dr. Daniel Siegel "is a kind of focused attention that allows us to see the internal workings of our own minds," I created shifts in my own attitude, while trusting a greater unknown, and I visualized light at the end of the tunnel (Siegel 2021).

Seven months later, a wiz of a young surgeon at Massachusetts General Hospital, Dr. Dahl, took out my ureter and clipped my bladder laparoscopically. For a few moments I was worried that it might leak or break. He convinced me not to worry. I remember having had a similar moment of panic when my left kidney was removed. How could I live with only one of them? My primary care physician at the time had said, "No worries. That is why God gave us two—just in case one doesn't function well." I wasn't completely reassured; giving up body parts and having your insides rearranged is unsettling. Grief showed up like a blanket of very dense fog.

It took another year of recovery before I could function somewhat normally. I had acquired chemo brain in the form of memory lapses such as forgetting people's names. I also acquired neuropathy in my extremities. Sprinkling cayenne pepper powder in my slippers helped to some extent. Native Americans are known to do this in order to keep their feet warm. I have always had an affinity for the nations who had handed down their practical knowledge and sacred wisdom. When I was a kid, I had imagined myself as a scout somewhere out West, on beautiful and glorious land, living with some benevolent tribe. Fantasy or not, it felt real and brought comfort.

After three years of being disabled, I thought I was ready to go back to work, in some function or other in healthcare, the field I knew best. I sent out dozens of résumés and over the course of one year I landed just four interviews. I was in my midfifties, with a varied skill set and a history of high salaries, and I knew that in the interviewers' eyes I was a financial and emotional liability. A friend of mine, who was a healthcare consultant, advised me to tell people truthfully why I had not worked for a period of three years.

During interviews, I realized that my mind was like gelatin as I shared the reasons why I had been out of work for such an extended period. As soon as I mentioned the Big C, they were eager to thank me for sharing such sensitive information, told me how much they loved my skills and experience, and how deeply my story touched them. Then, they shook my hand feverishly, telling me in a hurried way that they would call me back very soon. It felt like I had contracted Ebola, or the plague, as if they were fearful of becoming infected. One thing about patients who have been lying in bed, keeping our own company, is that we know immediately, in our gut, who is ill at ease, toxic, or inauthentic.

I knew my phone wouldn't ring. I had been on the upper management side of business, the executive director of a specialty hospital and other systems, and I knew not to bring in damaged goods. Nobody wants to hire someone who cannot be relied upon for long-term employment, someone who might be cost prohibitive, depleting insurance funds and requesting too many paid sick days. I got very depressed, realizing that now I was free of rogue cells I had very little purpose or usefulness in this world. I was running out of money from my savings account. Taking my Volvo and driving 130 miles an hour into the big tree down the road, seemed like an efficient way to get rid of the rejections and subsequent depression. It occurred to me, however, that I might end up paralyzed from the neck down, since Volvos are supposedly indestructible. That was enough to change my mind about suicide as an act of courage. Making choices to stay free of rogue cells was a better way of fostering bravery.

Eventually, a colleague who had worked for me a few years prior connected me with a headhunter, and I got an interview date shortly after. I went to Boston with no expectations, going through the motions, pretending to look for work. But life provides unexpected twists and turns. As soon as I let go of trying too hard, a position manifested. I probably uttered three sentences during the meeting and landed the significant position of Marketing Director on the spot. I went happily back into the familiar territory of corporate healthcare.

I needed the money, connections, and challenges. It was a real challenge at first, crunching numbers, working with new colleagues, traveling within three states, attending lots of board meetings, and taking part in regular conference calls. My chemo- and molasses-muddled mind did slowly recover and became an ally once again. I functioned well after a year or so.

Unfortunately, after three years the company was bought out by a much larger one. I was in a troubling situation; my position was a perfect fit for me, and the company operated like a family business. I prided myself on being the last corporate person from the previous management group to be let go. I had not yet figured out how to step out of my comfort zone when necessary. It took another three years before I left healthcare, saving some money in the meantime, unsure what I was going to do next.

I found both my vocation and avocation with Roshi Joan Halifax, Abbot and Founder of Upaya Institute and Zen Center in Santa Fe, whom I had met often in New York City and Western Massachusetts over several decades. After my illness, she said, "Come to Santa Fe, sign up for the chaplaincy program. I believe this is your calling!" I entered the Buddhist Chaplaincy program, graduated, and became ordained as an end-of-life care chaplain. The training was outstanding, led by inspiring and diverse faculty members. St. Martin de Tours, patron saint of chaplains, cut away half his coat for a homeless person, wrapping himself in the remaining half. The word "chaplain" is derived from the relic of St. Martin's cape. The legend is an important reminder that we can offer care to others without neglecting our own well-being. Practicing self-care, we recharge with physical exercises, artistic endeavors, meditation, singing, or having another passion or hobby that takes us beyond our worldly, conventional notion of self.

I joined a group of social workers in organizing yearly weekend retreats at Mount Holyoke College, where families affected by cancer could come and participate in all kinds of workshops such as kayaking, energy healing, massage, and easing or navigating the burden of financial and legal issues. These retreats were uplifting and brought some respite and time-out to caregivers, showering them with good food, physical exercise, and physicians' presentations on all types of cancer. It was a place to receive and give tender, unconditional love and compassion among a group of dedicated volunteers and professionals who had recovered from cancer.

I have been serving as a chaplain in hospitals and cancer centers teaching mindfulness practices for people of all ages, ethnicities, and economic backgrounds for the past thirteen years. When I lived in Western Massachusetts, I was asked to join a group of palliative care physicians from different health organizations to discuss cases and how to improve patient-centered care. Together we explored how professionals from many disciplines could communicate more efficiently about patient issues and better facilitate care. There was great cooperation between all the professionals from various health systems seeking and sharing ideas about how to best serve their patients.

For the last two decades, I have provided workshops on organizational management and development. Rogue cells are present in the context of corporate, nonprofit, and government agencies that lack strong leadership. I offer talks, workshops, and plenary presentations to individual clients, companies, physicians, and other clinical staff about end-of-life care issues and principles. I also teach people how to be truly present, proposing solutions for untangling the snares that prevent us from making the most of this precious life. I am on a most rewarding journey and have the privilege of coming together with amazing people on the path to recovery, with its many fateful twists, some troubling and dreadful, some marked by fun, copious laughter, and profound insights. I am constantly filled with gratitude, vividness, and lucidity from observing and sharing the many ways in which the mystery of life may be embraced and how we may honor the transition into the next world.

PART TWO:
ATTITUDE

Assault

The body is your nearest environment.

—Jean Klein

The assault of rogue cells in the body, prior to learning about the dreaded diagnosis, is an invasion of mostly silent, alien elements that undermine the natural functioning of the patient's body. For some people, the cancer is well advanced at diagnosis; for others it is in the early stages. Regardless, the trajectory of destructive cells running amok needs to be explored, assessed, and stopped, if possible. We all have cancer cells in our bodies that remain dormant. Usually, patients want to know what precipitated the activity of the cells that broke through their retaining wall.

The rogue nature of cancer is influenced by a myriad of variables, and so is the process of recovery. The extent of the cancer journey differs from patient to patient. The diagnosis of a stage IV transitional cell carcinoma was for me incomprehensible. My body was under siege and had been so for a while. My want of an explanation as to what had activated the initial, rapid progression of my cancer became a lifelong quest for information and enlightenment. This pursuit has involved in-depth discussions with oncologists and other doctors, including my son who is a multiple-organ transplant specialist, countless hours of research mining books and articles from various disciplines, and, of course, fervent introspection.

Through my work with cancer patients, I have gained a deeper understanding of the lives of cells and the interrelationship between the body, the mind, and the various levels of human consciousness. By supporting others in open, honest discussion and self-exploration, I have objectively witnessed dynamic effects in cases of essential life transformations. In this chapter, I concentrate on the biological workings of the body and share the knowledge I have acquired, in order to lay the foundation for you to develop strategies for overcoming emotional and spiritual barriers to your own natural healing process.

Cancer Cells as Rogue Agents

Let's look at the lives of cells and their functions. It is key for us to understand their role in our health and illness. We'll explore the functions of normal cells first.

- They differ from their parent cell and gain a special identity with a specific purpose, which causes them to gravitate toward other cells with similar functions.
- They are shoulder to shoulder with other cells, making proteins.
- They develop specialized tasks while belonging to a colony and contribute to the overall functioning of the larger organization.
- They communicate with each other and are part of an interdependent network in which they regulate each other's growth, behavior, and health.
- They only propagate offspring that have the same functions as the parent cells, and they are very cooperative rather than competitive.
- They know when to die. Regular cells have a gene for self-destruction; an evolutionary and altruistic, built-in program.

Now, we'll look at the lives of cancer cells. When cancer cells invade one's body like terrorists invading a foreign land, we need to understand their malignancy, intentionality, and directionality. Cancer cells are rogue agents that create anarchy and don't self-regulate. They are like a truck without brakes rolling down a hill, accelerating toward chaos.

- They don't have the capacity for self-definition, which means they don't mature or evolve.
- They do not specialize or work for the greater common good of the colony.
- They are not connected to reciprocal networks that might influence their growth and behavior.
- They co-opt the normal cells' ability to form blood vessels that help heal wounds.
- They divide and reproduce uncontrollably.
- They don't exhibit a higher motivation or harmonious purpose.
- Their telomeres, the enzymes at the end of chromosomes, are shortened.
- Their DNA becomes sticky and the protective elements collapse.
- They reactivate telomerase in adulthood, evade the immune system, and create their own blood supply.
- Their last function is to kill the host.

From an evolutionary perspective, life has moved from simpler to more complex forms of expression, and there is now more tension between individuality and conformity. On a cellular level, the drive for uniqueness is preserved, because differentiation is vital to survival and development. Taking a cue from the life of cells, when you value your identity and strive for the purest version of yourself, you can make sense out of what might seem unimaginable and unmanageable. You can effect positive change and support your being—not just your body—in the midst of extreme circumstances.

It is curious to me that there are algorithms to diagnose cancer but, as far as I know, none to eliminate cancer cells. Similarly, the mystery of the striking split between healthy cells and rogue ones has intrigued me. There must be some way to harness the energy, force, or drive behind the breakthrough of rogue cells, by holding a vision in mind that favors positive opportunities and wholesome outcomes. Rogue cells are unresponsive to the needs of others and create their own separate organism with no regard for the whole. They have little to give and lots to take away. Having poor boundaries, they tend to invade the space of their neighbors. They are not capable of learning from experience and have very little insight. Reactive, not connected with others, they operate without responsibility or responsiveness to any group.

Interestingly, they possess a lot of stamina, ostensibly derived from an absence of purpose beyond invading or taking over. This intractable grit wears out the larger organism, which they must infect in order to propagate themselves. They replicate forcefully. Then, opportunistic infections are met with limited resistance from a compromised immune system. Cancer cells are certainly exploitative, and like any deadly pathogen, they will take advantage of a debilitated host.

It is quite possible that these rogue cells are inspired by unconscious elements or unresolved patterns. When I was newly diagnosed, I wondered if it was conceivable that the cancer cells had taken advantage of me because I had not followed my own values. Maybe I had not fulfilled some call, dream, or vision, and settled for less than what was possible. Was the speed of cell proliferation commensurate with the number of unconscious states of avoidance, resistance, or possible constructs counter to my beliefs and values? Was there a lack of transparency? I needed to ponder some of these questions to be invested in my own healing, possibly prevent cancer cells from going rogue, and halt their homicidal trajectory. As my cancer had materialized amid my career disenchantment and the ruins of an affair that traduced my own moral code, it was not unreasonable to associate the propagation of the disease with the presence of hazardous thoughts and ideas. After years of reflection and analysis, I can acknowledge that I had jeopardized my integrity and my immune response concurrently.

Cancer is not one disease but rather a collection of diseases comprised of cells that have become perpetrators due to internal and external changes and genetic mutations acquired over time. Changes or mutations in the genetic material of normal cells are due to interrelated factors that are biologically based or exacerbated by lifestyle habits, internal and external stress, exposure to toxic chemicals, tobacco, improper diet, excessive and direct sunlight, and other environmental risks. The burden of these irritants, sustained either voluntarily or incidentally, disrupts the balance governing cell functions, which may lead to cancer.

Hormones, proteins, and nutrients also influence the development of cancer cells. These compounds and substances stimulate the growth of blood and lymphatic networks that supply the cancer with required oxygen and nutrients, which in turn allow them to move on to other sites and organs: this is metastasis. The immune system can identify and eliminate rogue cells, but often this system is suppressed, which allows the formation and progression of tumors. Chronic inflammation will weaken the walls of immunity around cells and promote cancer cells to develop and move toward vulnerable parts of the body. Carcinogenic mutations lead to a proliferation of defective cells which become tumors (from the Latin *tumere*, meaning "to swell.")

Researchers often measure the success of chemotherapy in relationship to whether a tumor shrinks, and by how much, which doesn't necessarily reflect an improvement in outcome. Other plausible factors involved in the success of treatment are the emotional and mental components of stressors: depression, loneliness, trauma, abuse, unhealthy behavioral habits, addiction, and a lack of a spiritual outlook on life. Over time, these factors significantly wear down the obstacles that keep intruder cells at bay.

The promising news is that there has been a steady and significant reduction of cancer deaths since the 1990s, according to the American Cancer Society (2019). More research has allowed for clinical trials, molecular targeted therapeutics, and immunotherapies. Even though cancer rates have been slowly falling, several million more cases of cancer are projected for the year to come, and cancer remains the second leading cause of death after heart disease. Universities, drug companies, governments, and philanthropic organizations have allocated generous funding; the National Cancer Institute alone has spent billions of dollars since former president Nixon initiated the "war on cancer" in 1971. Any war lasting this long deserves some reconsideration of our basic premises for its potential causes. Fortunately, much progress has been made on the prevention side in the last decade.

Still, we have more questions than answers. What events lead a healthy cell to become a cancer cell? Why do some parts of the body become impacted rather than others? What is the relationship between body cell mutations and cellular abnormalities? Can the force of habitual and dysfunctional thoughts and behaviors dominate us and tear down defenses that preclude insurgency, thereby allocating power to the rogue cells that feed on rigidity and chaos? Our search for answers within ourselves and from our collective resources is in itself an empowering stride toward a future where anxiety and uncertainty are stripped of dominion.

One July evening, on my way home on a backroad, there was a person walking frantically under an ominous sky with lightning flashing, and thunder rumbling. I stopped and asked him where he was headed. He had no idea. I realized he was homeless and asked him to step in the car. I planned to give him a ride to a used bookstore with an adjoining coffee shop next to a waterfall not far away. I thought he would benefit from a hot coffee. Suddenly, the storm raged. He asked if he could stay in the car for a while. I agreed of course.

He said, "Today I'm lost, totally lost in so many ways. You know, I had severe pain in my right side, to the point where I couldn't sleep lying on it. I found out this morning that I have liver cancer. I'm completely lost." He started crying.

After a long silence, he continued, "I'm very sorry to bother you with this . . . thank you for stopping and picking me up . . . listening . . . what can I do? I don't have any insurance. I'm lucky I can talk with you, I've usually taken pretty good care of myself, but with what I need, I might as well be dead now! This is unreal!"

I finally spoke: "I'm going to take you to a shelter and take a different road. I know the staff there can put you up for the night and help you get medical support. I know what it feels like, I've been through a cancer journey myself. You will find a way to get through this if you take care of yourself; if you get to the point of believing you can. Will you promise me to follow through? I'll call the shelter tomorrow and make sure you'll be guided in the right direction." I gave him resources, phone numbers, talked to the social worker of the residence, and dropped him off.

Weeks later, I heard that Michael had followed through and received chemotherapy at the local community hospital. Two years later I went to a music hall where he was working at a show, in a small college town. He filled me in about all the changes. He was in remission, had stopped drinking, attended AA meetings regularly, and made enough money to rent an apartment and live on his own. He had found himself and chosen a better path. He called me each July for two years in a row to say hello and let me know he had found a purpose for living and thanked me and many others who didn't give up on him. His recovery, as described, was a real struggle. He kept grounded as best as he could and later on found a way to make drastic lifestyle changes with a remarkable attitude.

I want to share a meditation at the end of this chapter, called space meditation, that helps us focus on keeping the mind big and spacious, preventing us from unraveling or being hijacked by negative and despairing thoughts.

SPACE MEDITATION

Just sit comfortably in a chair or cushion and breathe normally. Count to three on the inhalation, three on the pause, and three on the exhalation. Repeat three to five times.

Let go of the counting and notice the space around you, above you, and below you. Notice the space inside your body, inside your hollow organs.

Notice if there is any space between your last thought and the next one. Every thought has a feeling tone. Notice the space between your last feeling and the next one.

Now see how the space outside and within you has changed. What hasn't changed is the quality of your attention.

Now just observe what appearances of the mind arise: thoughts, desires, memories, projections, wishes. Notice the beginning, the middle, and the end of each phenomena rising and dissipating.

There is nothing to hold on to, nothing to push away, just be aware of the changing elements, coming and going.

There is nothing to eliminate, nothing to illuminate.

Whenever you space out, use the breath as an anchor to stabilize your body and mind. Wherever you go, you can connect with it.

Keep your mind big and spacious!

Terror

Fear is the cheapest room in the house.
I wish you would find better accommodations.

—Hafiz

In the time between diagnosis and treatment, terror is inevitable. It is a turbo-grief and sorrow that paralyzes us. We cannot get around it, we must go through it. In most people's minds, cancer is synonymous with life ending abruptly, causing terrible physical and emotional hardship along the way. People rarely expect to be diagnosed with cancer cells and certainly dislike surprises that hint at life suddenly coming to a halt. The state of shock accompanied by a loss of meaning and dignity, without an immediate strategy to overcome the problem, is daunting to say the least. I had been in strong denial for many months, knowing that something serious was altering my body, but I was reluctant to find out what was going on.

My familiar world changed drastically with this short statement from the oncologist: "You have a stage IV aggressive cancer." I was overwhelmed by the unimaginable. There was no place to land, at first. When reality eventually hit home, I attempted to figure out what options were available in order to make peace with this unwanted reality. For most of us, it's difficult to process complex challenges, radical change, the paradoxical, or the inconceivable. Even if we have shown compassion to a family member affected by cancer, and many of us have, one thing is certain: no one wants to catch it. There is nothing to be caught, of course, but maybe everything to be released.

When a patient receives their diagnosis, they often slip into a temporary state of amnesia or shock. Then questions arise abruptly. Why me? Why now? What did I do wrong? Major physical and mental disorders take time to develop and produce symptoms. The diagnosis, however, propels the patient immediately into a no-man's-land of unfamiliar and scary territory. Beliefs and ideologies are suddenly tested; the meaning of life and spiritual and religious convictions are questioned.

Patients fear that we are never going to be our familiar selves again. And it's true enough, we never will. The ego has a preference for certainty over uncertainty, predictability over surprise, control over chaos. When the rug is pulled from under our feet, there is no solid ground to stand on, no reference point to grasp and hold on to.

Whatever our response, diagnosis generates turmoil, suffering, and dread. This book's opening image of the conflicted body-in-suspension, hanging from a branch by the teeth, is poignant because it calls attention to our shortcomings. If we have not been awake or aware of what is meaningful or purposeful during our illness-free lives, we have limited comprehension of our existence. But at the doorstep of our potential demise, we are propelled into accounting for our usefulness and what we might leave behind after the final act in the theater of living.

The finality of life without an exit clause is a deeply disturbing notion. When either chaos or rigidity surfaces, we feel stuck and are unable to accept impermanence, loss of control, and liminality. The perception of self suddenly loses its firmness, and it feels as if everything is temporarily suspended and meaningless. American physician and neuroscientist Paul D. MacLean's often-referenced model of evolution attributes instinctual behaviors and primitive drives to the reptilian component of the triune brain. This structure is especially active in fight, flight, or freeze states. Disruptive emotions, including aggression, ensue when we are confronted with threats to our safety and security.

A patient without mindfulness skills or contemplative experience receives a cancer diagnosis as a frontal assault that dissolves all notions of normalcy. When we don't know how to pause, relax, or move information from the reptilian complex to the frontal cortex, which cools the bottom-up-activated neuronal jets, we are unable to make sense of the trauma. We experience "shock and awe," except there is no awe, but rather an overwhelming stage fright that immobilizes us and renders us speechless. Emotional self-regulation, which allows us to manage information and stimuli, is crucial to navigating the brain's neuronal axis, an imaginary line moving information from the reptilian brain to the frontal cortex and back down to the reptilian brain, to calm the central nervous system. Being aware of what is going on in this oldest and most active part of the brain allows us to pay attention to what goes on in the amygdala, which is capable of calming the mind by integrating the information in the rational area of the cortex. This process reduces agitation and lessens anxiety. And it requires practice.

STOP

I teach a practice in my mindfulness classes that is very important for calming the mind and making it serviceable. It is called STOP. We adopt this simple acronym to move from autopilot to drop into awareness and allow change to unfold when we are emotionally aroused.

- "S" means that we Slow down. Stop all activity. Do nothing!
- "T" stands for Taking deep breaths, many breaths, to bring Tranquility to the body and mind.
- "O" means we Observe, with Openness, our sensations, feelings, and thoughts, whether they are pleasant, unpleasant, or neutral.
- "P" means we Pause, holding the experience in awareness, and proceed when we are calm and can respond to whatever or whoever has upset us.

This acronym can be a lifesaver, giving us the opportunity to delve into our wholesome, natural capacities to align with our core values. Then we can interact with others in a safe, productive, and healthy manner. Use STOP to remember that there is always an opportunity to slow things down, particularly when you are least likely to be kind to yourself, or anybody else for that matter.

This practice came in handy to manage emotional dysregulation when I was sick. The acronym also helped me tremendously during my days of clocking 40,000 miles a year for business without completely losing my mind over spaced-out people on the road, talking on their phones, not yielding the left lane, ignoring the rules of the road, or driving with all the comfort and gadgets of a living room on four wheels. Of course, my righteous indignation made things worse. I am in recovery now and don't drive as much anymore. I remain hypervigilant when I do, as people are more absentminded than ever, multitasking behind the steering wheel. When driving, let's just drive. When involved with any task, let's just focus on it.

PANIC

Panic frequently follows the initial shock of the diagnosis. We wonder what to do with the many pills we've been prescribed, who will really support us and how this journey will end. Motivational imbalance grows, as we have very little energy to engage with others and follow through on plans. Or we simply shut down. Emotional balance is hard to come by and we may have drastic heart rate variability, living between fear and hope. We can easily go from a hyper- to a hypo-arousal state, obstructing homeostasis in our bodies. As we endure treatments, grieving is natural, considering the sheer number of multidimensional losses. We lose body parts such as breasts, kidneys, lungs, or bladders. The chemo side effects produce neuropathy, and steroids keep us up all night. We feel like damaged goods and especially unattractive. Cognitive dysfunction—difficult moments of trying to remember what we were going to say, the inability to integrate information to make plans or resolve simple issues—constitutes a full-fledged brain fog. We lose sight of what day it is, except for the dates we need to see our oncologist or attend procedural appointments. Those stand out like flashing red lights on our calendars.

We have a difficult time figuring out who we are now that we don't work. We feel unfit to contribute to our communities or the world at large in the way we had before. Playing a functional role becomes absurd, as we lose touch with colleagues, relatives, friends, and often partners who cannot bear to slow down and who may be worrying about their own mortality lurking around the bend. Improbably, we find ourselves suddenly lacking communicative filters, saying shocking things, suffering memory loss, becoming a complete stranger to ourselves and those around us. But each one of us is responsible for eliminating our own fears from one moment to the next, along with the major, constant irritants that create anarchy in the body and the mind. It is necessary to find and explore healing avenues toward basic wholesomeness on this unfamiliar journey.

Laurie is a stellar example of this. She was born in Japan and came to the US with her mother when she was seven years old. She got married young, had two children, and divorced when they were five and seven years old. Her mother helped her out while she was teaching at a large university in Massachusetts. When she joined the support group, diagnosed with stage III kidney cancer, she was on sabbatical. She never told her colleagues at work about it. Some cancer patients do; others choose not to.

She was shy and worried about work, her children, and especially what the outcome of her illness would be. She was exhausted all the time, lonely, and at the point of giving up on life. Her ex-husband had left her for a younger woman, and she had hardly recovered from the betrayal.

The support group was very beneficial for her. It allowed her to open up and share feelings she had never expressed before, about her estrangement from her culture, her mother's lack of ability to show emotions, and the academic world, which wasn't her real community. She'd always wished to be a businesswoman, owning apartments and selling real estate.

She connected with me because we'd received a similar diagnosis and my being in remission gave her some hope. She enrolled in the eight-week mindfulness-based stress reduction class I was leading and started to regain confidence in herself, smiling more often and releasing pent-up emotions about her abusive marriage and her children's absent father. Letting go of many destructive emotions in a safe manner was healing for her. In her culture, there was no platform for that. It was certainly impossible for her mother to express her feelings.

When Laurie's chemo regimen was complete, she felt hopeful about her dream of starting a real estate business. Her face lit up as she talked about it; she was ready to move on and live a new life. After three years of treatment and changing her outlook on life, she was cancer-free. She kept coming to the support group to encourage new members to believe life was worth living. She offered rides to those who needed treatments, in between her real estate appointments and sales. She was grateful for her new lease on life and gave other cancer patients the gift of staying involved, modeling her recovery behavior, and believing in unlimited possibilities.

Laurie initially experienced terror and worried about what was going to happen to her children and her job. The support group, and the mindfulness-based stress reduction course, helped her to make supportive changes on many levels. Becoming more aware of her internal life, paying attention to wholesome strategies, and following an intention to move toward managing and regulating her emotions served her well. Her vision to follow her dreams of a more rewarding job that utilized her strengths helped her find meaning and purpose.

Jeanne didn't fare as well. Originally diagnosed with breast cancer, she found out five years later during a yearly visit with her primary care physician that she had metastatic ovarian cancer. She was a very gifted and creative French woman, who made beautifully embroidered coats and colorful hats, while managing a used bookstore with many special, unusual editions. She gave me an out-of-print book of comparative idiomatic expressions in English and French, called *Le Coeur sur la Main*, that to this day makes me laugh and ponder how some of the unusual metaphors were created. For example, the English idiom "to be a black sheep" has the French parallel *etre une brebis galeuse*, which translates literally as "to be a scabby sheep," producing quite a different image in the mind. The literal translation of the title is "the heart on the hand" but the English idiom is "to wear one's heart on one's sleeve." Offering someone your hand with your heart in it is a powerful and precious image. It would have meant so much to Jeanne if her father had managed to do that. He was abusive when she was growing up, and she learned that it was okay to unleash decades of repressed anger on others.

In the support group, she would often give free rein to her anger about her dismal predicament of cancer recurrence. Sometimes she misdirected it at members of the group who were in recovery from cancer, throwing unexpected curve balls with an intentional smirk. She would apologize afterward. I often had to coach her in the group meetings to help her find more wholesome ways to express her frustrations. Yet, she skillfully modeled how to welcome deep, clear emotional insights and receive what others needed to say with pointed concern.

She and I met separately a couple of times and became close; maybe we both missed our birth country's language, and the companionship was comforting. As she drew closer to the end of her life, she found solace in accepting her lot, and I appreciated her will to do so with grace. She consulted a therapist to make sense of her predicament and tried to regulate her temper. Early childhood trauma made her strong in many areas of her fast driven and exciting life but also held her hostage in her emotional world, which was predominantly ruled by anger. She was willing to make changes that would bring her peace of mind, and she was successful at experiencing it more often. The illness moved faster than the adjustments she attempted to make and took advantage of her because she was exhausted by it. Fortunately, she was able to release some pent-up emotions, slowly but surely, before her departure.

Her husband shared with me, after she died, that she'd apologized to him for often being unavailable and bitter. She died peacefully in his arms, finally free from building walls, harboring resistance, or wallowing in resentments. I was content to hear that she left us without remorse. Surprisingly, she gave a generous donation to the cancer center in my name. It is such an honor to have been in her and her husband's presence.

The Meditation on Fear: Friend or Foe demonstrates how fear can be a catalyst for change if we refuse to become immobilized or pretend it doesn't exist. Fear has strong energy that we can harness and benefit from. Knowing we don't have to identify with our feelings is freeing. We can have moments of elation or distress that don't affect our deepest essence.

MEDITATION ON FEAR: FRIEND OR FOE

Fear is part of being human and, although it is not comfortable, it can be useful. We are wired to respond to fear negatively but need to make friends with discomfort temporarily.

Where in your body can you feel it? Breathe awareness into different areas. On your outbreath, release any constriction.

Repeat until you feel the release. Don't judge if you don't immediately feel at ease in your body, being kind to yourself will benefit you.

The raw energy of fear often gives us the élan vital for a fuller life and is neither good nor bad.

Exerting volition to overcome fright, or pretend it doesn't exist, does not send fear away.

Fear often produces great awareness, alertness, and vigilance that support us in intentionally changing a situation and making better decisions in order to respond to it.

Fear galvanizes us and allows for feats of strength we wouldn't otherwise achieve. Being at ease now, you can recall such a moment.

We don't have to live as if our hair is continuously on fire. Fear doesn't last for long when we are aware of it and release it.

Notice how fear and love are closely related. When we love, we fear for others.

We are grounded, we are not suppressing fear or ignoring its central place in life. Being blind to fear is far more dangerous than facing it.

Remember, feelings and thoughts will not last forever and are not the totality of who you are in any given moment.

Relax into your basic goodness, effortlessly. Your mind encompasses everything.

Trauma

Between every stimulus and response there is a pause, and in that space lies our power to choose our response. In that response lies freedom.

—Viktor E. Frankl

Trauma ensues from the sheer force of the unknown, the experience of loneliness, and being subjected to chemotherapy and other invasive, mostly toxic, therapies. To cope with the shock of a horde of cancer cells, you need to assess how wide your window of tolerance is. You need to protect your life force and at the same time face the notion of premature death, which is mostly unspoken of in our culture.

Answers don't come easily when we are in a state of shock. However, questions abound, and some will remain unanswered. In *Letters to a Young Poet*, Rilke (2013, 18) urges:

Be patient toward all that is unsolved in your heart and try to love *the questions themselves*. [. . .] Do not now strive to uncover answers: they cannot be given you because you have not been able to live them. And what matters is to live everything. *Live* the questions for now. Perhaps you will then gradually, without noticing it, live your way into the answer, one distant day in the future.

What benefited me was decades of past meditation practice, which gave me the ability to tolerate change in so many aspects of my life. I applied this tolerance ahead of coming changes, whether the shifts were in my family, my work setting, or the healthcare system, while remaining calm. Meditation settled me in the midst of chaos, allowing me to balance doing and being, and helped me operate so I could manage change before it controlled me.

For instance, I was successful at work because I figured out what trends were most likely to develop in the marketplace and planned accordingly. When managed care began, I proactively developed a referral base in Canada for patients who lacked services and providers for psychiatry, drug addiction, traumatic brain injury, and ventilator support. At the same time, I developed relationships with managed care entities in the US in the early '90s, letting them know that they needed our services, and we needed their support. This allowed our company to sign close to seventy contracts ahead of the competition.

When it came to changes in my own body though, I became frozen in time for weeks.

Most of us know about impermanence conceptually, but we dislike living through enforced change. I was ill and my body would either move toward well-being or decay. I needed to find and evaluate new measures to address my predicament.

THE SEARCH FOR ANSWERS

It is common to want to take action right away. Cancer is associated with the swift, fierce multiplication of killer cells, that spread havoc and take over the host. In reality, it can take years before cancer cells break through their retaining wall. Autopsies have occasionally revealed cancer cells that remained contained and did not lead to symptoms. Over the years, I have contemplated the variables that weaken the immune system and allow cancer to emerge. One predominant variable is the quality of the "store consciousness," as outlined in the Buddhist tradition. It plays a significant role because everything we experience, beneficial or not, is kept in a memory bank. These stored experiences influence our actions but are not necessarily known in the conscious mind.

My key focus after the initial shock was to assess how I could strengthen my immune system and the relationships that influenced it. What resources, besides invasive medical procedures, were necessary to move toward eliminating the cancer? Should I work with the physical issues solely? Or should I reevaluate my view of who I was and my relationship to the world at large? Should I integrate new tools to optimize being at ease in my body, mind, and heart? And if I could not be at ease in this body, could I improve my quality of life for whatever borrowed time was available? Could I move from obsessing about negative outcomes to foreseeing alternative options with sustaining qualities?

Any of these questions elicits more than one response, and we are unlikely to receive the answers instantly. The elusiveness of immediate relief is unsettling and creates panic, confusion, and a string of unpleasant thoughts. Simply breathing slowly can be a revolutionary act in the midst of rapidly evolving change. Pain and suffering can be managed with both medication and meditation. Meditation rarely has side effects, and is usually harmless, unless we use spiritual bypassing to forgo therapy and avoid dealing with emotional problems, focusing on spirituality solely as an escape.

The anguish brought on by drastic change is legitimate and most inconvenient. Grief washes over us in the wake of uncertainty, because there is a fissure between our expectations and what is actually happening. Change shatters and scatters our delusions about phenomena and experiences into a seemingly meaningless heap of unrelated parts of our lives. When our storylines don't make sense anymore, and the identity we have built around them vanishes, we need to release them. Yet we rarely do, because at least we know the outcomes of our miscarried plans, no matter how painful and disturbing they might be. The unfamiliar is, unfortunately, unwelcome in times like these.

Our former self-images no longer serve us when cancer cells blast away all illusions of order or firm constructs. This crisis of identity tempts many patients, unnerved, to undergo swift, unnecessary, expensive, and dangerous invasive therapies. I vividly remember a support group member, Nick, who was in the last stage of testicular cancer. His wife panicked and started calling specialists in faraway hospitals and research centers. But he was too sick to be transferred and ended up in a small community hospital one weekend. His bowels were blocked, a colonoscopy was ordered, and his colon was perforated in the process, which sent him into a coma. Then a tracheotomy was ordered. He died a couple of days later. He could have benefited from palliative care services either at home or in a hospice setting. Comfort care would have been provided and, more than likely, he would have been conscious and present with his family and friends before taking his last breath. Hospitals and prisons are rarely the first choice of place to die.

Preparation for death is important and warranted but, just like when it comes to taxes and wills, most of us believe there is plenty of time to "prepare" before the deadline. Nick passed away, like so many cancer patients do, in a hospital intensive care unit, receiving emergency interventions, instead of dying at home with hospice and palliative care services geared to put the patient at ease. Care partners, often with the best intentions, panic as they experience their own trauma. They look for swift, expensive, special interventions to help their loved ones, whether necessary and effective or not. Care partners who devote all their waking hours to an ailing loved one sometimes secretly wish the end would come sooner. We can't blame them. Being a care partner requires 24/7 attention and constant presence. Some patients live for years, degenerating slowly as care partners witness them turning stranger than any stranger.

For me, being sick and having to be dependent on others was the crux of an oppressive problem. Death seemed acceptable with comfort care but having to be taken care of by my children would have been a terrible burden on them. Some caregivers who crisscross the country when a catastrophic illness strikes also have the responsibility of making decisions that will effectively end their loved one's life. Nobody is ever prepared for that dismal task, regardless of the religious or spiritual beliefs they espouse.

WIDENING THE WINDOW OF TOLERANCE

On an emotional level, we all have a window of tolerance that informs our view of ourselves and the world in which we function. The width of this window varies in size for each of us. Let's imagine that the window is the shape of a cylinder. Any time there is a stimulus coming our way, we try to manage and make sense of it, keeping the information within the container. If the stimulus is too threatening, overwhelming, or highly challenging, we might not be able to integrate it. The information produces a hyperarousal or hypo-arousal state, and our emotions move up or down or even outside the container. The inability to manage information coming our way, unfiltered or unassimilated, creates emotional distress, moments of high anxiety or depression, and puts us way out of our comfort zones.

When we receive unknown, threatening stimuli and information, we often push them away or ignore them. Unfortunately, as Carl Jung said, "What you resist not only persists, but will grow in size." This popular expression applies to emotional energy because what we put off will surface at the least opportune moment and add more stress and suffering, due to unwanted change. We prefer to initiate change ourselves, but if that cannot be the case, we can invest in modifying our approaches and responses to it instead.

The influence of friends can be unpredictable, and while they often have good intentions, the outcome might not be favorable. Sometimes we need nice little white fences around us, because people whose neuroses are fully in charge of their lives suck the energy out of us. It is hard when we are ill to have to listen to other people whining about their minor discomforts. It's even worse to have to listen to unsolicited litanies of advice, suggestions, and expectations for what is of the utmost importance in "beating cancer." One of the issues that comes up frequently in support groups is that the patient, instead of getting reinforcement, is drained by the selfish admonitions of those who think they know best.

It is especially hard to deal with people who are suffering a lot and yet unwilling to change the narrow perspective of their outlook on life. In Buddhism, these wretched beings are known as hungry ghosts. They have narrow throats, are constantly in need of nourishment and are never satiated. They repeat the scenes of their misfortune continuously in the same act without the respite of a proper interval.

When we are ill, it is common to wonder who will meet us in moments filled with despair. Who can support us when we don't have much to say or share? We prefer to have someone to hold our hands. There are so many important things we are not taught about in life, such as practicing presence and how to intervene when someone is in need. I often wondered on whose lap I could rest my heavy head in the absence of words, tasks, or plans for the future.

Through introspection, we can determine what is beneficial or detrimental to the well-being of our minds. The more we can live in the present, the less we become overtaken by strong beliefs, uncomfortable memories, concrete judgments, and unrealistic expectations that prevent us from being in the moment. With a meditation practice, we can look at the relationship we have with appearances of sensations, thoughts, or feelings. The more spacious we are, the more we lessen our reactivity, and the less we space out or dissociate. Increased attention gives us more clarity and the possibility of modifying our intentions and actions in order to become healthier. Redirecting our attention from the surface level of the mind's many narratives toward the pure immediacy of the present moment allows us to break away from the trancelike ego realms, and this provides us with choices. A spiritual journey is a calling from the depth of one's psyche, whose source is timeless, sacred, and luminous, and we can feel this when our attention and intentions are working in sync.

COMING TO TERMS WITH IMPERMANENCE

> Everything flows, you cannot step in the same river twice.
> —Heraclitus

Why do people wait for memorial services to say wonderful things and share kind feelings and memories about their deceased partners, parents, children, friends, and relatives? Dead people will never hear, and might not have known, how they impacted and inspired other people's lives, or what great benefactors they were before being laid to rest or reduced to ashes. Maybe we've got it backward. Could we call it something else besides a memorial service? A celebration-of-life festival? You might come up with significantly better terminology.

Memorial services are primarily a celebration for the sole benefit of those left behind to grieve. This is important, of course; grief comes in waves and always lasts longer than the party. In fact, it shows up for years, often out of the blue or related to some unexpected memory. It is so important to let people know, while they are alive, how much we love and respect them in their deepest essence. We could all use practice putting aside petty concerns and complaints.

When we are in open awareness, called "suchness," we accept the reality of the moment. Instead of wanting this or that and thinking in terms of "should" or "shouldn't," and "could" or "couldn't," we might be able to relax, letting go of the burden of conditioned thinking and the old imprints that weigh heavily on us. There are ways, approaches, and methods that will allow us to maintain our integrity and guide us during the acute and unexpected phases of sorrow and suffering resulting from cancer. They begin with an acceptance of impermanence.

Everything is impermanent: flowers, buildings, political regimes, opinions, feelings, perceptions, relationships, views, and every mental construct. When a thought is observed, it vanishes as another rises immediately. This is not just an idea. The existence of anything is only possible because of the interdependence of everything. Nothing has an inherent nature of its own, and everything is always dependent on favorable causes and conditions to take form and exist.

Our feelings, thoughts, and sensations are ephemeral and elusive within the vast awareness of the mind. When we perceive continual change as loss, it creates the insidious, nagging feeling of missing out on something; a deep, underlying dissatisfaction. This weighty and overriding malaise makes us constantly wish for stability, and we adopt convenient remedies and instant solutions.

We spend a tremendous amount of energy viewing things as permanent, stable, and fixed, or perhaps wishing they were. Alas! What goes up will come down, what comes together will eventually come apart, and whatever is created will be destroyed. We primarily suffer because we wish for things to stay the same. Yet knowing that everything changes might encourage us to savor and cherish many moments of our rare and precious life. Dualism is very much alive in us and problematic. When we understand "suchness," the state of mind free from conceptual thinking such as labeling, analyzing, deducting, comparing, and making a point, we can accept impermanence more easily. We drop into our immediate experience, and our resistance to the present diminishes.

When we acknowledge impermanence, the desire for pleasure or avoidance of discomfort, the acquisition of things or fear of losing them, our looking for praise or wishing not to receive blame, and our concerns for our good or bad reputations, all lose their grip. With active cancer cells in the body, the pull of gravity not only shifts for the afflicted person but for everyone around them. Rogue cells destabilize any imagined sense of order, justice, benevolence, or status quo.

ACCEPTING MORTALITY

I am not afraid of death; I just don't want to be there when it happens.
—Woody Allen

And then there is the ultimate loss, coming face-to-face with the Grim Reaper, from whom we cower even though we know all humans die. We will leave for an unknown realm, naked again, without any belongings, letting go of this world we have barely come to know. We feel a sense of urgency to postpone the loss of our names, egos, personas, histories, and relationships. Simultaneously, we must relinquish the illusion of permanence. The drive to find remedies for fatal diseases is at odds with the noble wish to leave an immortal legacy. Death, which is incomprehensible at the rational level, is perhaps the biggest existential joke of all, considering that we learn a lot, make many connections, and accumulate things only to grow old and have to give everything up. Maybe we can even become wiser as we age if we take the opportunities to apply our learning.

Joe was the father of a reverend friend of mine, who belonged to the same clergy committee as I did. We supported the city, offering ideas on how to manage immigration, migration, growing substance abuse, trafficking victims, the growing homeless population, and the community's lack of adequate services. The father was an oncologist specializing in brain tumors. He became dizzy one day and lost his balance. Thinking he might be exhausted, he went home puzzled, somewhat concerned. The next morning, he fell. He immediately made an appointment with a fellow physician, who ordered a CAT scan. A couple of days later he was summoned by the doctor, who told him that he had two large tumors in his brain. Surgery was not a viable option, as they were lodged in the sensitive motor cortex. When the news got out at work, his staff found it inconceivable. His family and friends were also dumbfounded. He died so suddenly that everyone who knew him as a gentle and soulful mensch was profoundly affected and sad.

Joe regularly referred patients to one of my support groups. He was a great oncologist, specializing in brain cancer, but he wasn't prepared to deal with his dreadful situation. He isolated himself, only feeling safe around his medical team. He was not ashamed, but sadly couldn't face his helplessness and hopelessness. He was attached to the overarching concept of "I, me, mine." Although we are certain that we will not live forever, we all behave as if we will. A testimony to our insanity is that people—even wealthy and famous ones—regularly die without a will, leaving a legal mess for their heirs. Their money goes into the state's coffers, or the family members spend hour upon hour fighting for what remains after the lawyers are paid.

Being alive naturally involves encountering impermanence. Depending on how we meet it, we can find impermanence liberating or debilitating. If we yield to it, we claim the mystery of ongoing movement and stillness, found in the waves of the ocean and the rhythm of a heartbeat. No one can ride the crest of a wave forever—surfers know well that no wave is ever constant, and so do people living with illness. The biggest billowing breaker we will face is death.

When we let go of the fear surrounding our mortality, we discover, through contemplative practices, a way to embrace the tension between feeling and thinking, being companionless and in relationship, wanting more and rejecting what we have. Learning to relate to internal and external stimuli with equanimity, we appreciate the many gifts life has to offer and prepare for the one permanent and finite event to come. The path along the way is what matters, not the mysterious destination.

Such preparation helps us when the final, sometimes labored, breath arrives. It also causes less harm for those connected with us. I was shocked when I heard, years ago, that Dr. Elisabeth Kübler-Ross, renowned for her dedication to and remarkable work with the dying, didn't pass peacefully; her final months were spent waiting for God, "a damned procrastinator," to take her (Nolan 2002). None of us know how we will exit this life. The notion of a "good death" is one of our greatest aspirations and also one of our worst delusions. A life lived in peace with kindness and wisdom will often ease the transition, as I have witnessed with those who die gracefully.

MEDITATION ON THE 9 CONTEMPLATIONS

All of us will die sooner or later. Holding this thought in mind, I abide in the breath.

Our life span is decreasing continuously. Holding this thought in mind, I delve deeply into its truth.

Death will come whether we are prepared for it or not. Holding this in mind, I enter fully into the body of life.

Our life span, like that of all beings, is not fixed. Holding this thought in mind, I am attentive to each moment.

Death has many causes. Holding this thought in mind, I consider endless possibilities.

Our body is vulnerable. Holding this thought in mind, I attend to my inhalation and exhalation.

Our loved ones cannot keep us from death. Holding this thought in mind, I invest wholeheartedly in this practice.

At the moment of death our material resources are of no use to us. Holding this thought in mind, I exercise non-grasping.

Our own body cannot help us at the time of death. Holding this thought in mind, I learn to let go.

(From Upaya Zen Center, "Being with Dying" retreat, 2004).

Intervention

One doesn't discover new lands without consenting to lose sight of the shore for a very long time.

—André Gide

Intervention is necessary in a crisis of this magnitude. Calling on a sober mindset and letting go of unbeneficial habitual patterns, conditioned thinking, and core beliefs about ourselves, we reevaluate what will serve us best to restore homeostasis. We do need to rest after diagnosis and accept the news, but standing firm in the ground of being while doing nothing does not meet our needs at this stage. Now, we are invited to explore thoughts, affirmations, and core principles that will assist us and bring clarity. Our spiritual practice involves honoring life, waking up to larger realities, and seeing ordinary life as sacred and healing.

This may not come naturally. We are wired for drama, because we have a default mechanism in our hippocampus, that prioritizes any upsetting information and negative or disturbing feelings. These tend to lodge in long-term memory, while the particular details of pleasant moments dissipate within seconds. We can offset this habitual accumulation of strife by practicing breathwork and gratitude for being alive, to help curtail rumination, anger, and other unsettling emotions.

The body is a complex system, which as with any finite system, eventually moves toward self-destruction. Within it are other distinct systems, such as circulatory, respiratory, musculoskeletal, central nervous, and endocrine, that function in synchronicity, representing what we understand to be physical health.

Over time, some of the individual components of the body experience wear and tear. Then a profound discomfort and functional imbalance arise. Often, self-regulating elements are compromised by consistent external and internal inputs prior to illness or due to aging. When we are sick, our bodies are challenged to manage threats and inflammation, requiring tremendous energy for optimal functioning and restoring wholeness. In addition to the body, our emotional, cognitive, and spiritual worlds are complex. The separate components of our incredibly manifold being must work together to complement one another and function as intended. Like a mobile over a child's crib, when one piece moves, all the others will readjust their positions.

Having breakthrough rogue cells in the body creates imbalance. Any interventions we apply need to be assessed judiciously for the creation of worsening outcomes or additional problems. Too much chemo or radiation, for instance, can cause harm by depressing the immune system, lowering the white blood cell count, and burning tissue. Sometimes we don't know until the interventions are initiated whether the results will be constructive. Good intentions don't always produce positive effects, and multiple perspectives and approaches need to be evaluated and amended regularly. It is worth taking risks, and contingency plans are always warranted because changes abound all around and within us in perpetuity. Our inclinations toward positive change invite beneficial outcomes. We know our thoughts affect how we view and approach situations and relate to other people. Similarly, the mind influences and alters components of the body on fundamental levels, as we will explore in the following section.

EPIGENETICS

In many shamanic societies, if you came to a medicine person complaining of being disheartened, dispirited, or depressed, they would ask one of four questions: When did you stop dancing? When did you stop singing? When did you stop being enchanted by stories? When did you stop finding comfort in the sweet territory of silence?

—Gabrielle Roth

When our hopes for change dim during a crisis, these four questions are pertinent to consider. Dancing, singing, stories, and finding comfort in silence affect our physical and mental health because they bring us peace and joy and lift us above the daily grind. How we interpret our world is translated by the brain into chemical information that adjusts the behavior and genetics of cells to complement our perceptions. This is the theory behind epigenetic science as it relates to psychobiology (Church, 2014). The Greek root *epi* means "above," and the overarching meaning we assign to the events of our lives—mentally, emotionally, and spiritually—affects genetic activation. The quality of our consciousness influences and increases gene expression, causing parts of the brain to activate genes and change enzyme levels that are responsible for repairing the ends of chromosomes, called telomeres. The dogma of genetic determinism has been upended now that we understand genetic activity is affected by factors outside the cell, primarily through thoughts and our relationship to experiences and our environment.

Epigenetics looks at the sources that activate gene expression. When I lead mindfulness-based stress reduction classes I start the class by asking participants to share what they want to let go of and what they want to gain from the course. I tell them what mindfulness pioneer Jon Kabat-Zinn, (2012, 61) writes in his book *Mindfulness for Beginners*: "As long as you are breathing, there is more right with you than wrong with you, no matter what is wrong". Reminding people that they are more well than unwell is like turning on a light switch; time and again this simple testimonial has awakened inert sufferers and stimulated renewed energy.

Personal perception, lifestyle, and spirituality all can adjust genes to manifest either a functional or dysfunctional state. Siegel (2017, 184) maintains it's possible to "actually change your brain and the various molecular mechanisms underlying neural functioning and bodily physiology" by reducing stress and improving our responses to emotions. How we respond to experiences influences the expression of genes that stimulate the formation of new neurons. This gene activation is intimately connected with healing and immune system function and has a correlational relationship with consciousness. Unpredictability and novelty are important catalysts for learning and especially effective when one has been given a prognosis of four-to-six months to live. Richard J. Davidson (2012, 174) in *The Emotional Life of Your Brain* cites the myriad of research, including his own, confirming that our patterns of thinking can "alter brain activity in fundamental ways, enabling people to leave behind unhealthy patterns".

A steady meditation practice over the course of many years, culminating in several thousand or more hours, promotes high-frequency oscillations called gamma waves that build long-term traits such as peaceful states, loving-kindness, patience, altruism, compassion, and resilience (Church, 2014; Davidson & Begley, 2012; Goleman & Davidson, 2017; Siegel, 2017). Tibetan monks, after more than ten thousand hours of contemplative practices on average, show gamma waves activate as soon as they start their meditation. They drop into a baseline of peaceful states instantly, and they even retain this post-meditation.

When emotional changes occur in the psychological realm, the biochemical homeostasis in the body is affected and possibly disrupted. Biochemical states are the product of gene expression. Multiple published studies show the link between emotional states, gene expression, and immune system functions (Davidson et al., 2012; Siegel, 2017). Looking at the sources that activate or suppress gene expression and energy flow, we need to assess the quality of our consciousness, which has the capacity to boost or inhibit the passage of information along neural pathways. How we assign meaning to experience is one of the primary factors that affects which genes are activated (Church, 2014; Siegel, 2017). This interpretation of external stimuli, and our relationship to it, is especially crucial during periods of illness in order to reinstate homeostasis and balance.

DHEA is one of the hormones most commonly associated with cell repair. Stress from having been diagnosed with cancer cells increases the patient's cortisol levels and depletes the adrenals. The production of DHEA increases when cortisol levels are low, allowing cell repair to occur (Church, 2014). Attitude, positive self-talk, nurturance, altruism, meditation, occasional therapy sessions, and spirituality are instrumental in promoting a healthy level of gene expression and T cells. Mindfulness can help prevent inflammation and reduce certain cancers (Davidson et al., 2012).

No matter how sick we are, we rarely lose the ability to manage our thoughts and feelings and harness those which support vividness and aliveness. We have a degree of leverage over our own health and contentment that makes the difference between giving up and rising above challenges and compromised states. The first step toward harnessing this leverage is to listen carefully to our existing quality of consciousness.

GIVING THE INNER CRITIC A VACATION

If there is something you can do about a problem, why be frustrated?

If there is nothing you can do, why get upset?

—Shantideva

When we get sick, it is easy for us to turn inward and blame ourselves, identifying with the cancer. We are not our cancers. We want instead to save our energies and strengthen our immune systems by keeping our minds open and free of judgments.

Mateo came to the US from Colombia in the late 1980s, became a naturalized citizen, and married a woman he'd met while working on a farm along the Connecticut River. Sadly, his wife died in a car accident fifteen years into the marriage.

He remained single after his wife's death, taking care of his brother's widow who was mostly confined to a wheelchair. His only brother had died on his way to visit their mother in

Colombia. Matteo assumed that he was killed by some gang; his brother never got to see their mother, and his body was never found.

Mateo worked hard on his small farm and had help from university students who studied farming nearby. He discovered one day that he had thyroid cancer, after seeking treatment for severe headaches, weakness in his body, and dizziness while working the fields. He thought his symptoms were caused by the heat and humidity of unusually hot and muggy summer days. He was fifty-nine years old.

Mateo was a kind man who was very religious but not affiliated with any church or congregation. He lived a simple life and didn't have many friends. When he came to the group, he was sad and weary, wondering how his brother's wife would get help if the cancer killed him. Members of the group gave him support and resources and suggested he live one day at a time.

I contacted him when he stopped coming. He said he felt he was making other people sad with his life story, his mother's death, and his inability to visit her before she passed away. He was afraid the members would resent his presence. I suggested he come back and talk about it. He did and was surprised to hear that it was not the case.

He returned every other week for about a year or so, the progression of his cancer worsening. He decided to go back to Colombia to die and be buried on his ancestors' land next to his mother's grave. We raised some money and gave him a new suitcase and cane, because his gait was compromised. On the final day before his departure everyone was in tears, giving him big hugs, fully knowing this was the last time we would see him and hoping he wouldn't die in the hands of a cartel like his brother. A group member drove him to the airport, and off he went.

We never heard from Mateo again. We waited weeks for a card or letter, but we were glad we had helped him fulfill his wish. Our intentions were more important than any unknown outcome.

Mateo overcame several obstacles while living with stage III thyroid cancer. He figured out a way to come back to the group after he realized he was not failing its members. He also let go of his fears about going back to Colombia, even though his brother had disappeared. He decided he had lived his life in this country long enough and followed through, ignoring his inner critic, honoring his ancestors' lineage.

We all have a critic in our heads that is rarely satisfied and often confused. We give it a full repertoire of detrimental crystalized core beliefs that do not support us. We need to give this treacherous entity a vacation as often as possible; these internalized thoughts amount to too much static, interfering with our abilities to detect the more reliable signals of our inner sanctity. Most of us are very hard on ourselves and rely on guidance from broken records that don't fit the reality we face in a given moment. In our culture, self-disparaging mantras such as "I am not enough," "Something is really wrong with me," or "I am a failure," are predominant. Most other restrictive and inhibiting beliefs can trace their source back to these three. Daniel Goleman (2003), in *Healing Emotions*, recounts that the Dalai Lama was shocked to hear Westerners tell him about self-loathing and their tendency to blame their parents for their problems. In fact, it took him some time to comprehend and assimilate what people were trying to relate to him. This was completely foreign thinking for him and his people, isolated from the rest of the world by steep mountain ranges and high peaks. In Tibetan culture, respect and devotion to the elders and their spiritual beliefs were sacrosanct; it was unusual to blame parents for hardships.

Our identification with these black and white core beliefs isn't useful and will accord us no assurance. Judgments always create distance within us and between ourselves and others, often with the summation "Thou shalt not . . . !" The world has lots of grey shades. With discernment, we can audit these familiar recordings, which we adopted long ago in order to protect ourselves. They are only maps of reality, not reality itself. Personal admonitions separate us from our deepest, most basic goodness.

MEDITATION ON LETTING GO

Sitting comfortably, let the mind rest in its natural state. Relax your body, let go of tension, contraction, or any strain.

Allow yourself to open like space. Spacious, the mind remains clear; relaxed and loose. The mind is transparent and luminous, not clouded by any disturbing phenomena.

Consciousness is not confined to the head, body, environment, or any specific place. It is vast like space and encompasses everything. It pervades all.

Remain at rest, relaxed in this limitless state of openness.

Let go of dullness or indifference and stay in lucid awareness.

Thoughts are just temporary movements in the foreground of your consciousness.

Notice the gaps between your thoughts. They might be entry points into still, unfabricated, nonconceptual awareness, clear and fluid.

Within this reality, contractions and tightness fade naturally, and we discover a raw tenderness and the fragile beauty of life as a whole.

We realize then that our thoughts are rarely as solid as we might have imagined them to be.

Just like a mirror that only reflects whatever appears in front of it, notice whatever appearances of the mind surface. They don't shatter the mirror or modify the reflection.

Watch the flow of phenomena, without choosing to embellish pleasant ones or push away unpleasant ones.

There is nothing to eliminate or illuminate.

Just rest in the middle of awareness, relax, let be, let go.

Let be, let go, again and again.

NON-IDENTIFICATION AND CONDITIONED THINKING

Last night while I was sleeping, I dreamt—marvelous error!—that I had a beehive here inside my heart.

And golden bees were making white combs

And sweet honey from my old failures.

(From "Last Night as I Lay Sleeping," by Antonio Machado)

The mechanism for releasing and changing old patterns is called non-identification. Patterns are clusters of thoughts and opinions that might have served us well at some point in our lives but have a negative influence over time, creating ongoing suffering.

We recognize patterns when we notice incongruity between our intentions and what actually happens. Without pushing this away, or ignoring the temporary discomfort, we give ourselves permission to feel strong emotions and notice the familiar cycles. Decisively, we give them up. The word "decisive" comes from the Latin root *cedere*, "to cut." In this context, we cut the root of our unhealthy patterns, which is necessary for continuing growth, building a gentle rapport with ourselves and engaging with others.

When we let go of negative core beliefs during illness, we take a plunge into the unknown, which is a benevolent energy field. When we trust life as it unfolds, we gain freedom from our knee-jerk reactions of holding on to what is pleasant and pushing away what brings discomfort. Attuning to our inner knowing creates spaciousness. We can drop into this domain, uncoiling the inner grip of tension and limitations, relaxed and grounded.

This experience of affirmation was particularly evident with Sandy, a transsexual who was diagnosed with advanced prostate cancer after having surgery to fully embody the woman she'd always believed herself to be. She had suffered a lot and become financially destitute along the way. Depressed and lonely, she was convinced that those around her were uncomfortable with her new identity. Prior to joining the group, she'd mentioned she was anxious and fearful of being rejected. I suggested she give it a try and make her decision after the first meeting. I shared that I had worked for a healthcare company with inpatient services specifically for LGBTs in the '80s. I had put together an advisory board comprised of professionals who knew the needs of the LGBT population much better than I did; as a result, I had an increased sensitivity to many of the issues Sandy conveyed to me. I assured her that she would be surrounded by people who were primarily looking for acceptance in a supportive environment.

She joined the group with some trepidation but was welcomed by all as another unique person with cancer who had a goal to live better. After a couple of sessions, she began to actively participate with her deep voice, speaking freely from the vantage of her genuine self. She became very close to everyone in the group, revitalized by the prospect of being more all right that awry.

Our conditioned thoughts tend to be like the needle of a record player stuck in a groove, producing repetitive noise, not playing any harmonious tune. Moving the needle creates a new reality by encoding pathways in our brain, making it possible for us to manipulate the levers of healing on our own. Many people regain health through the placebo effect whereas those who choose a nocebo effect do not fare as well. Optimism, altruism, meditation, prayer, social connectedness, gratitude, and wholesome intentions are the conduits through which our consciousness influences our genetic expression. The brain inhabits the body, and the mind transcends the body, giving us the opportunity to eliminate any thoughts that would provide rogue cells with the authority and liberty to invade our bodies.

MEDITATION ON THE TWO WOLVES

A Native American elder was asked by his grandson how he had become so wise, happy, and respected and why people would commit such horrible acts as the 9/11 attack.

The grandfather said, "Each one of us has two wolves in their heart: a wolf of love and a wolf of hatred."

The grandson asked, "Which one will win?"

The grandfather responded, "It all depends on which one we feed each day."

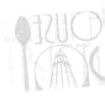

ADOPTING BASIC TENETS

> In the beginner's mind there are many possibilities, but in the ex
> few.
>
> —Suzuki Roshi

When my belly was cut open diagonally for the removal of my left kidney, and I v
several rounds of chemo, three tenets served as a rudder while I moved through da
waters. They gave me spaciousness, rather than fixed notions, around unfamiliar and
situations, and they were strong guidelines that matched my thoughts and feelings
my values and my innate North Star. They were my compass for a pro-social, gene
new beginning. The harm that results from unwholesome thoughts and behavior wh
basic standards of decency and morality can be devastating. Deep within my being
was wholesome and what was not. The tenets offered the possibility of a radica
threshold experience of undoing tight knots and, eventually, seeing the places I had
tenets I'm referring to are beginner's mind (sometimes called "not knowing" mi
witness, and compassionate action.

Beginner's mind teaches us to live fearlessly, consistently pushing methodologies and
opinions to the margins. We tend to analyze, judge, modify, and move away from experiences
which cause us discomfort, uneasiness, and anxiety. In supposedly protecting ourselves by
avoiding discomfort, we become contracted or immobilized. It requires quite a bit of energy to
make up storylines: the usual mental interpretations and superimpositions of concepts, ideas, and
biases about what we experience. Unfortunately, the process of creating the stories separates us
from experience itself.

We often become rigid when engaged in a continuous struggle, instead of interrupting or
breaking the cycle of our powerful agenda-drivers. If we allow ourselves to open up to what is, we
might become curious about our common, fundamental, profound humanity. We might realize that
in the most difficult and painful corners of our experience, there is always something fresh and
alive waiting to emerge for us. We might learn to yield more often.

Jody was a young woman in her early thirties who had a rare form of stage IV breast cancer.
She moved from Canada back to her parents' home in Massachusetts with her seven-year-old
daughter, after an abusive marriage and difficult divorce. She was sad and disheartened about the
rapid growth of the cancer cells, her looming death, and her daughter's uncertain future. One day,

while taking a short walk by the farmers' market, she met a man who owned an organic produce farm. She befriended him, finding him attractive. They talked often and he invited her out for a date. She was delighted and frightened at the same time. She asked members of the support group whether she should go on the date and open up to him about her illness. Group members supported her, in fact urged her, to accept the offer to meet him and be loved. She gave her inner critic a break and let go of all the "What if he doesn't stick around?" and the "What if I fall in love?" queries.

She went out to dinner with him, didn't eat much as her appetite had vanished quite some time ago, but had a wonderful time. She told him about her predicament, the journey ahead of her, and that there was no cure in sight. He didn't back off; they dated for a few months and got married before her illness worsened. She shared with the group, via conference call, her deep sadness about being loved unconditionally at this juncture and having to leave her daughter and husband behind sooner rather than later. She found moments of happiness in her declining days that she'd never expected or even dreamed of experiencing. Tears of elation streamed down her cheeks when she related her joy at being loved, even though her body was failing her. When she became bedridden, the group met at her house. She was grateful for the providence bestowed upon her, and for having followed the suggestions of the group's members, who rejoiced and found solace in her temporary happiness as if it was their own.

Her husband stayed by her bedside without hesitation and accompanied and held her on her way to the other shore. She was loved deeply and knew that he and her parents would take care of her daughter and help her grow into a beautiful being. Slipping into a brief coma, she died peacefully. Today, her daughter is an emotionally healthy eighteen-year-old. She wears her mother's wedding ring in her honor, never to be put in some dusty drawer and forgotten.

Jody, with stage IV breast cancer, learned to practice beginner's mind and lived in a formidable manner with the time allotted to her. She found solace in being loved unconditionally with heart and soul by her new husband and courageous daughter. The group's presence for her during this remarkable period gave her the room to be open, supported, and held in their hearts and wishes.

The second tenet, bearing witness, helps us go to the places that scare us within the territory of our tender hearts. Bearing witness develops our capacity to be touched and to be vulnerable. The word "vulnerable" evolved from the Latin word *vulnus*, meaning "wound." When we take the risk to open up and reveal our tenderness, we stand the chance of getting bruised. Bearing witness draws us toward intimacy with an instinctual pull; we are guided by our spirit. When present, we enter the relational field without any other goal than being fully available and holding space. This tenet is my principal guide in honoring patients and their disparate mind states.

The third tenet, compassionate action, allows us to become midwives, bringing things to the surface in a safe, gentle, altruistic manner. What motivates us is the desire to lessen our own suffering and the suffering of others. It is not about pity but our shared human vulnerability, giving us a nurturing stance. Nor is it about self-indulgence. Rather, it provides us with strength and resilience to meet anyone, whatever their position, in the midst of confusion. Empathy is not enough; we relax in our own or someone else's contraction, leaning into temporary discomfort, denying the tendency to move away from it or shut down. It is a kind, strong, and soft connected presence.

These three tenets helped me tremendously during my journey. When I was confronted with many questions I didn't have answers to immediately, not knowing was soothing. Bearing witness didn't require instant action or firm remedies, just active presence with other beings who were suffering. Compassionate action, without an evident fixed outcome, was the perfect prescription. Adhering to the tenets was the prerequisite to welcoming and cultivating equanimity, and they still guide me now.

Joseph, in his late fifties and newly retired, was diagnosed with stage IV esophageal cancer. His only son had been diagnosed with the same type, at stage III, five years earlier and had recovered after four years of treatment. Joseph hoped he would have the same positive outcome, but one year later the rogue cells invaded his liver. Practicing beginner's mind and compassionate action, despite tremendous suffering, he put his affairs in order, giving his wife and son all the details of the things he had taken care of around the house for years. He prepared for the inevitable, neither leaving things undone nor sowing confusion.

It takes a lot of stamina and intention to explore healing while struggling with exhaustion and reduced willpower. We benefit from inner work that produces new insights and provides clarity into the choices we face. These tenets are not just concepts; they are concrete, palpable, and applicable to our daily lives.

The Meditation on One-Pointed Attention helps us practice stabilizing the mind in the midst of unexpected change. If we had several animals tied together with one rope, such as an alligator, a monkey, an eagle, and a donkey, chaos would flourish. However, if each one is tied to a separate, distanced post, they won't go in all directions, fight, or kill each other. They will concentrate on being safe and safeguarding their territories. For the following meditation, the post represents our single-pointed attention, focused with stability and vigilance.

MEDITATION ON ONE-POINTED ATTENTION

The wandering mind is shaped by bodily sensations, sensory cues, and habitual thoughts and feelings outside our conscious awareness.

Its natural state is often uncontrolled, fixated on the past or future, and unaware of the present moment.

Placing your attention on the breath, which helps to stabilize the mind, hold your attention with steadiness. Whenever you get lost in thoughts, space out, or become hijacked, bring your attention back to the breath.

A quick and direct way to focus the mind is to count to three on the inhalation, three during the pause after the inbreath, and three during the exhalation. The counting keeps the mind steady with one-pointed attention.

Often, disturbing emotional states and unpleasant thoughts arise. These could be agitation, fear, turmoil, subtle yearnings, annoyances, irritations, discomfort, or recurring ruminations.

These can flare up and take hold for long periods of time or rage out of control.

Observe them without owning them, and then release them.

Simply experience mindsight. Use your attention like a telescope, focusing on your internal landscape.

With mindfulness we discover the ability to let go of biases, solid opinions, and judgments. Then awareness feels soft, tranquil, and present for the unfolding of experience. You are alert and have clarity.

Notice your attraction or aversion to phenomena, sensations, thoughts, and feelings, without favoring or rejecting whatever appears in your heart and mind.

Observe impermanence, selflessness, interdependence, and relatedness.

In this way you can gain an understanding of unconscious patterns deep in your psyche and transform them.

Realize that consciousness consists not of an unbroken continuous stream, but rather a continuum of brief moments of awareness.

Know that you are on the right track when your awareness rests in the immediate present and your attention is focused on the domain of the mind.

Simply note mental events or feelings that arise. Be at peace, keep your mind at rest, transparent, lucid, and spacious.

Mind states strengthened by kindness, compassion, generosity, and wisdom lead us away from suffering and, step by step, toward awakening.

Toll

A ship in harbor is safe,

but that's not why ships were built.

—John Augustus Shedd

The toll of cancer can be extensive: physically, emotionally, cognitively, and spiritually. Given the length and duration of the demanding cancer journey—from the activation of rogue cells to detection, prognosis, and the fallout from treatment—we are pushed smack against our sharpest edges: our fears that signal insurmountable danger, the unknown, exhaustion, yielding toward giving up. But this levy need not be a permanent roadblock on our earthly odyssey, leaving us stranded on the side of the road. In fact, though the cancer journey may be costly, grueling, and protracted, the bounty for moving beyond the devastation, and beyond survivorship, is immeasurable.

We must summon intense motivation to gather resources and new skills, such as the openness required to move beyond Velcro mind states that include feeling victimized and wishing to choose the path of least resistance. The evolution of cancer cells takes a long time from inception to maturity, ultimately resulting in a noticeable mass that may have advanced largely unnoticed by the host. Many people find out they have active cancer cells while going through a routine yearly checkup, or receiving treatment for some minor, unrelated medical condition. For some, however, the onset of symptoms comes as a surprise, like a lightning flash with thunder shortly after.

Such was the case with Henry, whom I met in one of the support groups. He was a college professor but not enthusiastic about his job. His real passion was for running long-distance races. He'd participated in the Boston Marathon to raise money for cancer treatment, because his son had been diagnosed with bone cancer. He finished the race in good standing, but the next day he felt excruciating pain in his abdomen. He went to see a physician only to find out that pancreatic cancer cells had already metastasized to his bones. He died three months later, having coped by smoking massive amounts of marijuana daily and isolating himself, except for attending the support group. He did not participate much in the group's discussions but was content to be among others who had "nasty cells," as he would refer to them, in their bodies. He had checked out. If he had applied his capacity for endurance racing to the long-haul course of recovery, he might have finished strong.

Cancer cells do not discriminate in terms of social background, age, or gender, but they do present a particular challenge for people who are not embodied. This means operating from the neck up and favoring Descartes' dictum "I think, therefore I am." When not fully embodied, we are inclined to believe that our thoughts are paramount and a manifest reality, rather than a subjective interpretation. We believe our awareness is primarily located in the conceptual realm of the thinking mind. Our contemporary culture tends not to emphasize gut awareness, or "felt sense," a focus on our inner, corporeal sensations. This paucity of full-body consciousness prevents us from recognizing when the physical self is under siege and ravaged by the side effects of constant stress.

Steady, constant stressors are the most dangerous kind. The chasm between what we think and how we act, together with a failure to release discomforting energy, creates an unsustainable physical environment like a pressure cooker about to blow its top. Here's an analogy used frequently in business circles and stress reduction programs: frogs thrown into a pot of boiling water will jump out, while frogs in a pot of water being heated up slowly will die. These unfortunate frogs highlight the danger of pent-up anxiety and tension that, when ignored, brings tremendous suffering. The more we are aware of the sensations in the body, the more we are able to respond to what ails us, what brings us relief from distress, and what motivates us to change.

It is not uncommon to have a difficult time feeling sensations in different parts of the body, because it takes practice such as trying yoga positions or listening to a body scan meditation to increase body awareness. Embodiment, although often neglected, promotes healthy functioning of the immune system, which we rarely consider as a critical component of health either when we are well or when we are sick and tired.

RELEASING TENSION

The immune system plays a wider role than just protection. One of them is to release tension and let go of the "issues in the tissues." Crying freely, without being pressured to "cheer up," allows human beings to suffer intensely while releasing body fluids, feelings, and thoughts. Painful emotions create the issues in the first place and plant seeds in the consciousness. Tears are a lubricant that facilitates deeper exploration of the emotional conflicts that have been created or adopted, without interrupting or sabotaging the process of discovering where we might be stuck or defensive.

Animals are much better than humans at releasing stress instinctually and have a wider tolerance for it. For instance, think of a bird on the ground who sees a big cat approaching. It will immediately fly up, land on a branch, shake off the threat, and move on. When we are stressed, we human beings will call our friends and commiserate about "the big cat," expecting them to acknowledge the awful situation, while they share their own outrageous encounters with big cats, exacerbating the incident. The stress remains, not only in the mind but also in the body. It is advisable to energetically discharge it.

The immune system, like consciousness itself, is not located in one dedicated organ and develops in response to challenges. A defensive response is only initiated upon the detection of an invading agent. The more we are able to release pent-up energy and strong emotions, the better the chance for the body and the immune system to relax and actually summon T cells that can reduce harm and stressors dangerous to the health of the body. Meditation, breathing exercises, body scans, and gentle yoga all actively support the immune system. Self-compassion exercises, kind self-talk instead of judgmental evaluation, and a loving connection with people who value altruism and empathy will help us become more pliable and experience a sense of calm.

A couple came to check out the group with ambivalence and hesitancy, unsure if joining would be a good idea and just wanting to get a feel for it. They lived way out in the hills on a sizable piece of land with no adjacent neighbors. Bill was a metal sculptor who made a living selling his art pieces to large companies. He had been diagnosed with bladder cancer, stage III. Ellie was also an artist, known for her water paintings, handmade poetry books, pretty landscape cards, and chenille scarfs and hats. She had been diagnosed with bone cancer in her left knee, which eventually metastasized to her spine. The diagnoses came as a double whammy, just weeks apart, and represented certain doom for the two of them, who had chosen a quiet life isolated from the "outside world." They didn't have much faith in the medical system, had no children or close family members, and wondered how this all might end.

Research has shown that one significant component of well-being, besides insight, purpose, and meaning, is being connected to a community, just like healthy cells working together for the greater good of the colony. The only connection Bill and Ellie had to their greater community was through the occasional sale of their art pieces. They might have been satisfied with their solitary lives, but during this crisis they decided to engage with others who were experiencing similar suffering from a common adversary.

After their initial visit, they decided to keep attending the group. They were glad to meet other people who had cancer, were on a similar journey, and whose bodies would possibly betray them sooner or later. Words didn't come easily to them, as they were used to solitude during most of their waking hours, but they attended faithfully for a couple of months until Ellie got sicker. Bill wasn't faring much better; he was in constant pain, having bouts of incontinence, becoming unmotivated and deeply depressed, unable to finish any of his sculptures that he had promised his patrons. As they became weaker and driving became more difficult, I set up a couple of group conference calls so they could attend remotely from their landline. A month later we found out from Bill that Ellie had passed away in the yurt, with palliative care treatment consisting of a constant regimen of morphine and other strong narcotics. Then, we had no more contact at all.

Eventually, one of the group members saw Bill's obituary in the newspaper. He had died a couple of weeks after Ellie and was found dead in the yurt by a kind neighbor. Their land was willed to the State as a wildlife and animal refuge center. The group learned from their example how crucial connection is, how important it is to show up for oneself and others, how to get up and not fold into depression, and how important it is to open up and keep trying to resource oneself with suggestions from those who are a few steps ahead on the journey. Often, group members share about beneficial choices they made and a how bit of encouragement provided wind to their sails.

OPENING UP

We have multiple possibilities with which to meet and relate to what is presented to us. At first, there are usually sticking points, repetitive internal summations that keep us from moving forward, a kind of arrested development, when we encounter challenges or catastrophes. For example, some caregivers fall away, unable to bear the loss of intimate moments and sexual pleasure. Eventually, we will mourn the professional care partners so devoted to us while we were sick, who leave us when we are in recovery. We are expected to return to normalcy, but we miss their companionship and compassion, as if another umbilical cord has been cut.

As we discover our capacity to open up, we eventually discover turning points that allow for new shifts. In Tibetan Buddhism, the three dimensions of being, the ego, humanness, and being fully human, are fascinating ways to understand how we may relate to our internal and external worlds. They can be compared to three different qualities of water: ice, still water, and flowing water.

The ego dimension is like water in the form of ice. It has sharp edges that can wound us. It is outer presence, past history, persona, and how we like people to perceive us. It is a functional and reactive self, focused on survival and primitive coping mechanisms. It is self-representational and has the capacity to formulate a consistent self-concept out of various images of self. The tragedy is that we start to believe these images and self-representations, and then we have to reinforce them over and over. It is strengthened by the conceptual dualistic mind, governed by fixations: "You are there, I am here." It is like a fortress that has the beneficial qualities of predictability, rigidity, form, and protection.

The next dimension is humanness, the relational self. Now, the ice is melting. We take ourselves less seriously and are open to realms of exploration and insightful activities. We form bridges with people and see relationships between matter and spirit. We cultivate a sense of adventure and move easily into fresh arenas and around obstacles. These are all water aspects.

Being is the third dimension, which relates to unobstructed, flowing water, allowing for continuous and diverse "flow states." This is the essential self: pure presence, openness, the world of "creating no separation," not losing sight of where the body, or mind, leaves off or begins. It is characterized by wisdom, fluidity, unconditional openness, and boundlessness with steady movement and stillness. Stillness is the source of love; movement is the source of life. To move and be still is being fully alive!

Cancer diagnosis affects our identities because the ego, primarily formed out of fixed self-representations, panics about loss. The tightness resulting from the constant need for security and control sets up a divide between self and other. Ego is like a closed fist. A hand permanently clenched suggests stasis. When the hand opens, it is possible to overcome the fear of giving up whatever it holds and receive whatever is bestowed. One method of catching monkeys in South Asia involves placing a banana inside a box with a small hole, big enough for a monkey to get its hand inside. When the monkey grabs the banana, its hand turns into a fist. Unwilling to loosen its grip, the monkey is captured.

A nurse, suffering from breast cancer, came to one of the support groups. She had been diagnosed with breast cancer a few months before retiring and was very bitter. She was obese, with high blood pressure and diabetes. Her diet was loaded with sugar, and she never took much time for vacation. She struggled to focus on herself in the group. Her heart had been broken when she was in her twenties, because her then-boyfriend was chronically unfaithful and dishonest. She never recovered from it. Food and work became her sources of nourishment, and she made sure to make herself look unattractive so that she would never be betrayed again. Over time, she learned to be kind to herself and set up new priorities. She did recover from cancer and a few years later eventually married a kind man and invited the group members to her wedding.

As the nurse realized, it is not impossible to change deep-seated patterns, and she eventually warmed up to the idea of the dimensions of ice melting into flowing water, moving away from resistance toward healing. The positive and nurturing self-talk she learned and adopted from the support and suggestions of the group members helped her to assess what degree of leverage she had over her health and contentment.

Malignancy is rarely affected by physical states only. Emotional obstructions are also a factor. There are therapy services that offer safe platforms to release emotional "stickiness," a translation of the Tibetan word *shenpa* which refers to our association with unpleasant experiences and the frequently detrimental coping mechanisms we develop to deal with them (Chödrön, 2019). The divestiture of *shenpa* combined with allopathic interventions tends to work well.

There is an inspiring story of two monks that illustrates *shenpa*. One morning, on their way to collect alms and food, an older monk and a young novice came to a river whose banks had swollen overnight because of the monsoon rains. A woman sat on the ground nearby, distraught, unable to cross the river to go to the market and sell her vegetables and fruit.

Out of compassion, the older monk offered to carry her to the other shore. He dropped her off on the other side of the river, then went back to carry her bounty to her. The woman was very grateful and offered them some fruit, after which both monks left.

They walked toward a distant village and collected some cooked food from generous villagers. After a couple of hours, on their way back to the monastery, the young monk, beside himself, unable to hide his distress and disbelief, said to the older monk in an explosive manner, "I can't believe that you touched a woman! It goes against our most fundamental precepts. How could you?!" The older monk responded calmly and said, "I dropped her off a long time ago. Why are you still carrying her in your mind?"

When we experience *shenpa*, it is as if we are standing in the train station, letting our train of thought move on, only to find ourselves time and time again riding the same locomotive, somewhere far away and disconnected from the present moment or situation. We tend to hold onto thoughts and emotions for hours, ruminating and mulling things over ad nauseam, dropping into a state of righteous indignation.

It is a daunting challenge to keep moving and let go of what we are holding onto dearly, even when it is counterproductive. There are risks from taking steps as well as from not taking any, and one important lesson on this journey is that we cannot afford to give up on living during any moment available to us.

MEDITATION ON ADVERSITY

Let's transform the mind so that even during adversity it becomes a friend and deep contentment abides in times of both hardship and felicity.

We have a conceptual mind and a perceptual mind. The former focuses on the past and future, not dealing with the present moment. It is busy interpreting reality instead of experiencing it. The conceptual mind is a "thought junkie," constantly planning, evaluating, comparing, deducing.

The perceptual mind is usually overwhelmed by all the concepts. It quietly attends to sensations without ongoing commentaries. The more we are embodied, the more we notice mental afflictions, such as anger, arrogance, craving, delusion, fear, and jealousy.

Self-centeredness makes your problems seem huge and other people's problems insignificant. Self-centeredness is a habitual—but not inherent—element of the mind.

Check your perceptions to find out if they are accurate. Ask "Is this really true?" Investigate the stories you tell yourself and see how they lose their power as you realize that things are not for or against you.

You are not your cancer, nor is it punishment for something you did or did not do. Circumstances are always neutral; your relationship to them is what makes them attractive, repulsive, or ephemeral.

In the face of fear during this challenging journey, remember your innate safety and touch your intrinsic worthiness and inner nobility, not by chasing after another moment but by opening up to the whole experience.

We resource ourselves with this simple contemplation:

I am safe in this moment.

I am well resourced.

I know what I need, and I can ask for what I need.

I am connected with others. I am not alone.

We may repeat these affirmations during seemingly adverse times as often as needed.

Understanding

The Thorn in the Heart
I discern here a thorn,
Hard to see, lodged deep in the heart.
It is only when pierced by this thorn
That one runs in all directions.
So, if that thorn is taken out,
One doesn't run, one settles down.

—Buddha

Once we understand that there are posttraumatic growth possibilities and realize that peace of mind can be found within, we can adopt a new vision. We do this by exploring our internal geography, improving our emotional intelligence, and finding humor and meaning in experiences beyond self. This brings relief.

Understanding demands that we look at information coming our way and attempt to make sense of it. This requires integrating knowledge to favor posttraumatic growth, by observing the different parts of the triune brain and their respective functions. The approaches I offer here subsequently allow us to make better choices and move forward toward well-being. In this chapter, we will look at how cancer patients who cultivate emotional intelligence, favor a hobby, or have passionate interests heal with a sense of purpose. Laughing is very good medicine, and watching comedy is a healthy distraction, taking us away from lamenting about our temporary discomfort.

I remember Jon Kabat-Zinn, saying at a Zen Peacemakers' conference in Montague, Massachusetts that "healing is being with what is." "Being with what is" suggests that we meet our edges squarely, without fanfare, and look deeply into our relationship with ourselves and our present circumstances. It is as if a thorn keeps repeatedly bruising the heart, letting a few droplets of blood escape from it. The thorn in the heart doesn't break the heart, but we want to remove it to create more spaciousness. This keeps us from becoming contracted and rigid in our thinking, and invites us to step inside the opening. The heart is a symbol of radiating love, when we can put aside our many negative thoughts. Fluidity, discernment, and openness do not compromise the natural defense mechanism of the immune system. Quite the opposite is true. A core protective duty in our complex mechanism of healing is to ward off intruder cells while pursuing homeostasis. As we repair any emotional state, the body is free to go about its essential functioning.

We can regain solid footing and stand firm in the central axis of our being—no matter what happens—when we realize that peace of mind and contentment have little to do with external factors. Cancer cells disturb the self-organizing processes and linkages between the differentiated elements of the mind, heart, body, brain, and central nervous system. We need to find the natural pull toward increased awareness, balance, growth, and healing. It doesn't come easily and in the midst of disturbing circumstances is very much an extraordinary feat.

Meditation is an important vehicle to calm our body and mind. It suggests that we "come home" to ourselves again and again, because the mind's busy chatter keeps us from listening with present awareness. Awareness has a mysterious quality to it that rests below the surface of consciousness. It is always present, even when we are caught up in the doing mode, and never battles with the mind. As explained in *The Psychology of Awakening*, the Latin root for "meditation" as well as "medication" is *mederi*, which means not just "to cure," but also "to measure inwardly" (Watson et al. 2012). It is a practice that brings us focus and attentional skills we can use to gain insight into our relationship to sensations, feelings, and thoughts without reacting. Meditation allows us to respond to stimuli with clarity and lucidity, while making shifts to live a wholesome life.

Patty, a Jewish-Buddhist practitioner and professional photographer from Santa Fe, was a superb artist and a dear friend. Her meditation practices were instrumental in helping her move beyond the personal self. She was very involved in her work, and she shared art shows and contemplative practices with many friends, who were her community of choice. She had published photography books of women and dwellings in Yemen, a Muslim country, where nobody had minded her presence for several decades. Her passions, before and after she was diagnosed with cancer, were opera, theater, and movies. Illness didn't stop her spirit from loving beauty and its many expressions. She busily attended many art events and was gladly received in so many venues. She flew back and forth to Paris, where she had an apartment and practiced Zen meditation actively with a small community. Her art and her meditation practices helped keep her alive for three years longer than the prognosis handed her by her oncologist .

VERTICAL INTEGRATION

Let's take a look at how we can make sense of information that comes our way and manage it for well-flourishing. The brain is not only under the skull but has bilateral pathways throughout the body. Regarding distinct parts of the triune brain model, the oldest component of the brain, often referred to as the reptilian complex, is situated above the brain stem. The limbic component is toward the middle, and the frontal cortex, the most recently developed part, is located in our forehead area. The brain has over 1.1 trillion cells and a 100 billion neurons that fire anywhere from five to fifty times per second. The brain, only 2 percent of body weight, uses 20–25 percent of the body's oxygen and glucose.

In *Mind* (2017, 137), Siegel writes extensively about top-down and bottom-up processing, referencing both the regions of the brain and the "distinct ways we experience the world". Vertical Integration describes the prefrontal cortex's method of sifting, sorting, and staging "the internal flow of sensations [rising] from 'below' into our cortically mediated awareness 'above'" (Siegel 2017, 92). In other words, we have the choice, through attention and awareness, to move the "hot, intense" information to the frontal cortex to make sense of it.

The amygdala hub is like the Grand Central Station of threat detection. It is able to discern uncomfortable and dangerous external and internal threats. It typically responds to stimuli with incomplete information. There are situations when our instinctual responses are adequate to deal with danger, real or perceived. For example, if a child is running into the street with a truck barreling toward her, we only need to know that immediate action is necessary to prevent tragedy; additional analysis would cause a critical delay. Under less dire circumstances, when we are not paying attention our thoughts and feelings can be easily hijacked. The amygdala hub is influential in creating automatic and usually unconscious reactions to stimuli, which become habitual or impulsive patterns over time. The neuromodulator for that area is norepinephrine, which functions to arouse and alert. There are a lot of fast neural-reactive responses and hot, emotional charges leading to passionate motivation that make up this part of the brain. This is why we might stay on high alert when dealing with the shock of a cancer diagnosis, which may hinder healing. We need to learn to calm our systems down through meditation.

The mesolimbic pathway is relationally driven and focuses predominantly on positive reinforcement, pleasant and unpleasant emotions, and feelings. The primary neuromodulator here is dopamine which relates to rewards and gratification. Too much dopamine generates an approach behavior whereas too little dopamine begets depression. Remembering that we need to stay connected with others—our brains are wired to be relational like our hearts and minds—helps boost health-related endorphins.

The cortex is the most progressive part of the brain and functions like an airport control tower. When confronted with multiple new phenomena, it determines what needs to be analyzed, compared, defined, assessed, and exposed. The key neuromodulator is serotonin, which regulates mood, sleep, and digestion, lessening depression and fear. This area is governed by the anterior cingulate cortex hub, which guides voluntary attention, allowing for emotional self-regulation and self-awareness. It is driven by will power, intentional choices, discipline, and metacognition, the capacity to "know that we know we know." It has a knack for simplifying complexities and takes us out of survival mode into healing potential. Empathy is primarily driven by mental, cortex-controlled processes.

This explanation of vertical integration is a primitive way of interpreting complex neurobiology. Looking at it through a three-dimensional framework is a much more accurate way of seeing the relationship between the elements of the triune brain. The point here is to realize that we have a neural highway or neural axis that we can use to cool the jets of the very active, hot, and concentrated components of the brain. We can move information "bottom-up," into the prefrontal cortex, thereby assessing ways to respond beneficially, rather than being governed by circumstances and involuntary, reflexive behavior.

If the emotional material that surfaces is not managed by mindful practices, or mindsight, the refractory period resulting from emotional arousal will last for long periods of time. With anger, for instance, if we are not aware of it in the body early on, it might turn into a wildfire, consuming us for hours, days, or possibly months, which will result in unwanted physical problems. The more we pay attention to our emotions and become aware of them before they take on a life of their own, the better the chance of not being held captive by our sentiments. If we drop judgment and shift our intentions, we can lessen the refractory time and release feelings in a healthy manner.

VASE BREATHING MEDITATION

The Vase Breathing Meditation was a secret practice handed down from teacher to student for Tibetan Buddhist practitioners. It was only revealed in the last few decades to practicing westerners. It has many benefits for the body and mind.

In this specific practice, we breathe deeper than in the diaphragmatic breathing methods often used in yoga. As you breathe in, imagine you are drawing your breath down to an area about four finger widths below the navel, a little bit above your pubic bone. This area is shaped like a traditional bud vase. As you turn your attention there, you will find you are inhaling a bit more deeply than usual and will experience more expansion in the "vase" region. This exercise moves energy beyond shallow, thoracic breathing that restricts energy flow. As you exhale slowly and completely, you will find your abdominal muscles move close to the spine.

Lung, is the energy force in the subtle body, where emotions emerge and abide, asserting a tangible effect on the physical body. Your *lung* will travel down and begin to rest there. It is a kind of intermediary between the mind and the body. We have channels and pathways through which this energy force moves like a wind. There is no movement without *lung*. It flows through the subtle body, carrying the spark of life which conveys the vitality that sustains our physical, mental, and emotional well-being.

Just breathe slowly this way three to four times, exhaling all the way down into the vase area. After the third or fourth time, try holding a little of your breath, maybe 10 percent, at the end of the exhalation. You maintain a bit of *lung* in its home place. Keep this up for the next ten minutes. In the beginning it might feel a little uncomfortable, but it will give you a sense of calm centeredness.

If practiced for ten-to-twenty minutes every day, vase breathing becomes a direct means of developing awareness of your energy and learning how to work with it in your daily activities. When our *lung* is centered, our bodies, thoughts, and feelings gradually find a healthy balance. Anxiety, anger, restlessness, and fear gradually loosen up when *lung* moves through the body.

EXPLORING EMOTIONAL INTELLIGENCE

Many people have heard of emotional intelligence, while very few people ever have a class in it. People compare their IQ levels with trepidation in our competitive culture, rarely considering emotional intelligence levels, which exhibit strengths or weaknesses that move people in favorable or unfavorable directions. According to Dr. Daniel Goleman (1998, 317), emotional intelligence is "the capacity for recognizing our own feelings and those of others, for motivating ourselves, and for managing emotions well in ourselves and in our relationships." This was very important for me, as a male, to explore how my emotions influenced my behavior and that of others. In our culture, little has been brought to men about how to identify feelings other than anger, which usually has accompanying underlying sadness. Exposure to a range of feelings is important for discerning intuitively what is going on in our emotional geography.

During my years working in corporate healthcare, I would interview people who had just graduated with a master's in business administration, thinking that their technical skills would be beneficial, which they were. Their relational skills were sorely missing, however, and their emotional states were rudimentary. I often had to let them go because they were unable or unwilling to adjust to colleagues and subordinates, or to collaborate.

The model of emotional intelligence, according to Goleman (1998, 26-7), is based on five competencies applicable to oneself and others:

- Self-awareness
- Self-regulation
- Motivation
- Empathy
- Social skills

In a workshop of Goleman's I attended, he divided the various aspects of emotional intelligence into two categories, one dealing with personal competencies and how we manage ourselves, the other about social competencies which determine how we manage relationships. This helped me relate all these competencies to the cancer journey and how to navigate it more efficiently.

Regarding personal competencies, the journey invites us to cultivate self-awareness, the capacity to read our own emotions and recognize their impact. As self-awareness develops, we gain an accurate self-assessment by evaluating our strengths and liabilities and checking our confidence levels regularly. When ill, it is very difficult to have an accurate sense of oneself, and often liabilities take the front seat in the thinking mind. Self-regulation allows us to monitor disruptive emotions and reduce any lack of impulse control. We learn to practice transparency and integrity, demonstrate adaptability, and overcome obstacles with enthusiasm and optimism. While undergoing treatment, many destructive emotions, such as anger, despair, or deep sadness, appear out of nowhere. It takes monumental steps to adapt and take the initiative to consider favorable outcomes.

Concerning social competencies on this healing journey, we rely on maturity, social awareness, sensing our own and other people's emotions, understanding others' perspectives, and being of service. Social competencies are about discerning how we commune with ourselves and others, resolve disagreements, and build a web of relationships through cooperation. We are reminded that we are not alone but wired to be connected with our fellow beings. Any emotion can be an opportunity for growth or a source of suffering because of its self-validating force; the principal source of emotion is love.

Whenever we close ourselves up to feelings, we have an attitude of stoic indifference, or emotional arousal, or dissociation, or passionate explosion. We can notice and shift our mindset, and this is an important healing choice. Below are samples of some of the most familiar and inhibiting emotions, the impulses they awaken, the opportunities they create, and the dangers that can lie within them. I relate these for the purpose of showing how they might impact people with catastrophic illnesses.

Fear

In general, we feel scared when we think the possibility exists that something terrible will happen or has happened; that we will lose something we value; or that we will not achieve a particular desired result. Post diagnosis, the possibility of losing one's life to terrorist cells running amok seems obvious, as most people think of cancer as a terminal illness with a definitive reduction in one's lifespan. The thought of cancer cells invading our bodies gives rise to many deep fears.

Effective action means that we address the fear, investigate unfamiliar areas, and take all possible measures to minimize danger in order to protect what we appreciate and value. The benefit of responding to our powerful emotions is that we may mitigate the potential detriment of the feared event. This definitely prevents and reduces self-imposed suffering. If we don't respond, we experience enduring anxiety, feel out of control, and likely re-traumatize ourselves. But there is an opportunity for transcendence. We can find confidence in our safety under the care of competent and supportive professionals, family members, and close, caring friends.

Anger

Decades of the "war on cancer" were demoralizing. Now we wonder if we are going to live, regardless of all the progress and targeted interventions made for some types of cancer. This can create anger. Dealing with life possibly coming to an end—and handling it gracefully—is very difficult. Anger is a combination of fear and sadness, or the feeling of someone having done something they shouldn't have, violating our boundaries, or behaving inappropriately.

Acting responsibly prompts the self-confidence to do the utmost in defense of our values. If we don't respond, we feel victimized and harbor resentment, rancor, hatred, or indignation. We need to establish limits and preserve our ethics.

Maybe we can accept that we have done our best so far in life. Self-compassion diminishes the charge of anger and judgment. Some of us are not able to let go of anger post diagnosis. This weakens the immune system; holding on to anger too long is a dangerous predicament for our physical, emotional, and spiritual well-being. On such occasions, instead of promoting growth and humility, we are often stuck in pride.

Pride

We feel proud when we believe we've done something of value for someone else, or ourselves, and we derive pleasure through public confirmation of the personal image we hope to project. Pride manifests when we want to be seen as remarkable and truly special. Pride in individual identity calls for self-recognition and self-esteem and focuses both on being and doing. When we recognize and value our identities, we discover the ultimate foundation, our inner wealth from which we energetically face the challenges of life, illness, and death.

On the other hand, when we aren't proud, we end up living with a permanent feeling of dissatisfaction and self-devaluation. The consciousness we embody is far bigger than our self-limiting beliefs. Facing illness and death, we rarely experience pride because autonomy and self-esteem are difficult to come by. In fact, pride and shame are two sides of the same coin.

Shame

Shame is the fear of making public any information that counters the image we want to project. It usually involves someone capable of revealing information about us that threatens the image we aspire to portray. This makes us fear humiliation. Shame stems from self-devaluation, self-degradation, and the fear of not being good enough.

When we detach and realize that all shame is based on false identification, we discover a source of security and possibly serenity. When we are ill, it is very difficult not to feel shame. Often with a diagnosis of cancer, we tend to believe we are the cancer. There is shame in giving up body parts, and facing our mortality; it's a real challenge to see the unique beauty we embody, because we feel unattractive, defective, defeated, and deprived. It is difficult to believe we are wanted.

Desire

Desire is the equivalent of hunger, thirst, or getting rid of an intense itch. Wanting something we don't have is a double-edged sword: on one hand it generates great energy; on the other hand, we might do things we never would have done had we considered the consequences of our actions. As long as we pursue our desires in accordance with our values, inner peace will result. Trying to obtain what we want at all costs creates frustration, dissatisfaction, and indulgence.

We wish to live and feel better, gain more strength, and be free of harm from cancer cells. These desires and needs are honorable as long as we utilize sound strategies to meet them. We don't need to ignore or suppress them. On the other hand, living without guilt is a must.

Guilt

Guilt is always based on the judgment that we transgressed our own limits and caused unwanted consequences or harm. It calls for us to apologize because we are remorseful; otherwise, it is a waste of energy and tainted by narcissism.

When we ask for forgiveness, we restore our integrity, reinforce our commitment to our values, and reduce defensiveness. We remember there is always another side to any story. Doing the best we can, we develop self-compassion and, naturally, compassion for others. When facing sickness or the end of life, we can let go of guilt and express remorse, making sure to ask for forgiveness from whomever we hurt so that we can be at peace. It brings relief not just for the other person but for us, too.

These emotions all present themselves with strong life-force energy. We must complement our understanding of them with a capacity for critical analysis and the ability to reframe different situations. It is not always possible to truly enjoy what we have, while it is possible to truly enjoy who we are.

A woman named Ann, who was an academic adviser for a large school system, had been retired for just three months when she was diagnosed with stage IV lung cancer and given a few months to live. At the time she joined the support group, she was sad that she had never traveled to several countries she had always intended to visit. Group members suggested she make plans to go, fulfill her wishes, and be exposed to different cultures and vistas. So, she visited Ireland and Australia, and then kept going, visiting several other countries, taking advantage of the short window of life afforded her. She returned and recounted her adventures and made us laugh about the many funny experiences she had along the way. She was a pistol!

Meeting our needs rarely becomes a problem, but the strategies we use to fulfill them may or may not be beneficial. After a couple of years of hopping on trains and planes, she ran out of money. Fortunately, her daughter, who lived below her, was able to support her at the end of her life. She lived two and a half years after her wanderlust began, before she moved into the small hospice where I was on the board of directors. When officiating her memorial, I heard stories about her that I couldn't have imagined from the people who knew her well. For instance, during her illness she would stay up until the wee hours of the night blasting Metallica, dancing, and belting out her own words to the music. Who knew that this staunch academic adviser would have this shadow side exposed to her daughter and son-in-law, both having to plead every now and then for a quiet night? "Who knew?" is one of my favorite expressions; there is so much more to human beings than meets the eye. When we let go of the urge to judge people by their appearances, we discover so many unusual gifts, passions, predispositions, and temperaments. Pearls only exist because of the sandy grit in their oyster shells and the constant rhythm of waves bouncing them around.

It is important that we are conscious of our emotions and feelings and work with them, or we will suffer the cost of ignoring them. This consciousness shows us how wide or narrow our window of tolerance is. When we develop an innate sense of what is important, we are able to make better decisions for ourselves. That is a blessing!

MEDITATION ON EMOTIONS

Emotions can become problematic when we feel them as forces beyond our control, given their powerful energy charge.

It is as if we stand tall against a mighty wave hurtling to the shore, the outcome never favorable!

Maybe we can let ourselves feel, let go of judgment, not suppressing or condemning whatever is challenging.

Our range of feelings can go from sharp and intense to global and diffuse.

The intricate tasks of the senses, soft skin, brain, and nervous system are all structured in such a way as to let the world in.

Feelings are our responses to the world when it touches us.

When we acknowledge our triggers, the world opens up and we discover the intense rawness and tenderness of being human.

A fearless and powerful proclamation is this: any state of mind and heart is a condition we can work with and has a larger intelligence than we might imagine.

FINDING HUMOR AND HOBBIES

One way to release tension from illness is to laugh. This is an effective medicine, which takes us to places beyond self-concerns. Discovering simple distractions is a harmless way to move from ruminating about the past or future into a larger field of energy.

JJ was diagnosed with a stage III melanoma, located in his jaw, which created an aesthetic problem for him. It was an annoying location, easily visible to anyone who came in contact with him. He joined the men's cancer support group, and his presence was welcomed. He was eloquent, a master of the English language, and his quick, dry wit made everyone laugh and feel at ease. He joked, "No woman would want to look me in the eyes. Not that they did before, but now if they did they'd get lost in the big scar, and that would be the beginning of the end. I don't even stand a chance to be rejected by a woman anymore!" He'd never been married and prided himself on having been unattached to anyone in particular during past, better days.

He'd been in remission for several months by the time he joined the group. He loved to be around other men, who didn't care about his slight disfigurement. He had a healthy understanding of his emotional world and was unafraid to explore his feelings and how they affected him. He didn't take himself too seriously, and others found solace in the lightness of his approach to the ups and down of life.

He had joined a writing group, and his wonderful penmanship appeared in local papers, serving as a productive outlet for his anger against politicians and incompetent municipal systems. He loved art, paintings, and music. He started a mixed choir, with many members in recovery from cancer. In summer, they toured Massachusetts and Connecticut, raising money for several not-for-profit organizations. They sang old songs from the '60s, '70s and '80s. Sometimes they would go to nursing homes and assisted living facilities, bringing joy to the elderly, who became reinvigorated for a few hours, their long-term memories serving them well.

We got together for lunch every other month or so and talked about the stuff of life: what was most important to us and what was getting us excited about our hobbies and interests. We often joked at our attempts to become more mature. JJ is doing fine today, with over twenty-three years in remission.

Different people like different types of humor, and preferences can morph over the years. For me, the companionship of Jerry Seinfeld, Robin Williams, and *The Three Stooges* was a big help during illness. Years later, watching *The Three Stooges* with my grandchildren, the humor didn't register the same way with me, coming across as primitive and aggressive. It involved laughing at the expense of others who were getting hurt. It had done the job when I needed it, however, allowing me to temporarily forget about cancer.

Besides watching comedy, one of my favorite pastimes is planting herbs, medicinal and culinary. I have been interested in growing healing plants since I was a young child, and I studied herbal medicine for a few years. I love the "doctrine of signatures," which determines the healing qualities of herbs by their color, shape, and what type of soil they favor. Most of the plants I grow or pick have wonderful scents: rosemary, lavender, bee balm, diverse mints, thyme, sage, anise hyssop, holy basil, comfrey, lemon balm, lemon verbena, and so many more. They bring me great joy, attracting bees, butterflies, hummingbirds, owls, tiny bluebirds, cardinals, finches, swallows, mockingbirds, and other beautiful feathered creatures. My back yard resonates with an orchestra of soothing sounds that calms my mind.

I have always had an affinity for birds of all feathers. I loved jumping out of planes, moving freely through space, defying gravity, being birdlike until pulling the chute. Often, when lifting my head, my eyes will catch the sight of birds. I remember vividly lying in a meadow, looking up, and watching two eagles performing a daring show above the ground, moving down and around, dropping at incredible speed against the blue background of the sky. What I interpreted initially as a fight was in fact an elaborate courting ritual, as I learned later from a bird expert. They left no trace, but in my mind, I see them still.

Even while I was sick, the world around me felt very much alive and inspiring, everything having its place and purpose. At night, sleepless due to the many steroids in my body, I would listen to the owls calling each other from opposite hills. Somehow, I knew deep down in my soul that I was going to be fine. I knew in my heart that I was going to discover a meaningful path in the not-too-distant future, while the present faded like objects in the rearview mirror of a slow-moving car. This knowing, this felt sense, was as soothing as a balm on a raw open wound.

THE UNFOLDING RIVER OF LIFE MEDITATION

Let your mind be a gracious host amid unruly guests. Know it heals itself and unveils its own inner resources for well-being. Think of your experiences and phases during meditations as a nonlinear flowing body of water.

The first phase might be like a cascading river, with the mind wandering here and there. While in your wandering mind, your experience appears to be chaotic; thoughts rise without continuity, free to drift. We call it "monkey mind." Become aware of how active your mind is and how thoughts are connected to sensations and sensory cues in the body. You may find yourself daydreaming about the future and past.

The second phase can be like a torrent in a gorge. By cultivating attention, you start to discover a direction in the practice. Subjective experiences are interrupted by distractions, but a sense of continuity begins to develop. With a focused mind you notice thoughts, sensations, and feelings before you space out. You are able to place your attention on the breath and hold it with steadiness to harness the unruly mind. Periods of mindfulness increase and, while it is rough going and not very stable, your attention is forming and building. Twenty-five per cent of your practice is on concentration.

The third phase might be compared to a river with rapids. As mindfulness stabilizes, your awareness develops and increases. You become more relaxed and welcome the quality of spaciousness. It is as if the water flows quietly for a time, then goes over some rapids again and back to flowing quietly. We might notice unpleasant and disturbing emotional states, restlessness and turmoil, and annoyance at noise, recurring thoughts, or uncomfortable bodily pain. Afflictions can flare up, grab hold of your mind, and rage out of control. Boredom, a state of excess attention with insufficient intention, might develop. There could be a constant, conditioned need for stimulation. But the "monkey mind" is becoming tamer. Abiding calm and peace arise more frequently, and you know that you are on the right track when your awareness rests in the immediate, present moment.

The fourth phase is like a lake with waves. You begin to accept the rising of thoughts and feelings as the natural movement of the mind stream. Awareness feels softer, more tranquil, and clearer. You trust the continuous changes. You realize that consciousness consists, not of an unbroken stream, but rather a continuum of brief moments of awareness. Reactive emotions surface and you simply notice; then they dissipate by themselves. You notice aversion and attraction, without favoring or opposing what shows up in the moment. You drop into presence, letting go of ruminating thoughts and unnecessary concerns.

Finally, you might experience "wise mind," which is like the vast, deep, calm ocean, without waves. The mind rests with clear, stable, and undisturbed attention. You are now experiencing equanimity, the ability to let things be as they are. As soon as any mental event or feeling arises, it is simply noted. Thoughts are just thoughts, sensations are just sensations, feelings are just feelings. They lack their usual intensity. You know that you are more than these passing elements of your mind stream. Effort becomes effortless, mind and body are at rest with clarity, luminosity, and stability. Over time, with repeated practice, the mind and heart propagate traits of kindness, humility, compassion, and wisdom.

Dependence

Wherever you have dreamed of going,
I have camped there and left firewood for you.

—Hafiz

Dependence usually has a negative connotation, because it suggests some type of attachment to, or addictive behavior toward, thoughts, feelings, or substances. These can include unmovable beliefs and strong resistance to change, as well as drugs and alcohol. In this chapter I use dependence in a positive sense: a reliance on our inner strengths and capacities to grow, heal, and find comfort and peace of mind. This makes it possible for any one of us to cultivate clarity, insight, kindness, and compassion for ourselves and others as they join us on our journey. To live beyond coping, we need to care for ourselves by practicing self-compassion and basic tenets. It is not selfish to become resilient and seek out a community of support, but necessary for moving beyond the wounded self. One source of support can come unexpectedly from animals—pets, or creatures in the woods—and from the mystery of nature itself, speaking to us directly in a universal language of tender, caring concern and faithful presence.

Another source of support, boundlessness, which derives from the space element, gives us spaciousness, openness, and interdependence. Instead of clamping down and narrowing our views of life during the cancer journey, we can see it as an opportunity for changing mind and heart states. In this space of boundlessness, we realize nothing has any inherent existence in and of itself. For anything to take form, it needs another phenomenon to support it. A plant needs soil and sun to grow. Every human being needs nurturing from someone in order to feel alive and to thrive. Unconfined space has no defined boundaries; it is expansive, spacious, and freeing!

I knew when I was told about my narrow window of four-to-six months to live that any development is dependent on favorable causes and conditions to manifest. Everything, pleasant or troublesome, is interdependent and interrelated, whether we like it or not. I had to cultivate vividness and luminosity, seeing things anew. It was time to meet the self that is greater than its individual components and belongs to the larger space of presence, resolve, and adventure. There were no old roles left or special hats to wear, just chilling nakedness, relinquishing that which didn't give me room to breathe. It was time to try something new and delve into what I never wished for in the first place. I needed to nurture a dependence on inner strength—a reliance on my own insight—through meditation, attending a men's support group, having Reiki massages, and participating in events at a local cancer center, such as workshops, holiday events, and fundraisers, where I could invite and receive care from others under one integral roof.

What comforted me tremendously during the early stages of my illness, after I moved back to Western Massachusetts, was my relationship with a young racehorse called Chicklet. I lived in a barn-apartment above a dozen Thoroughbreds. Chicklet had just been born when I was newly diagnosed. After my left kidney was removed, I would walk down to the stalls and talk to her, feeding her lots of hay and the apples she relished. She would eat out of my hand, and she helped me get over my fear of horses. As an adolescent, I'd been thrown off a horse immediately after mounting. I stayed away from equines after that, until Chicklet.

She was stunning, with her pitch-black shiny coat. I developed a love affair with her to an extent that made the other horses jealous. She would let me brush her and always welcomed me in the barn with happy sounds, lifting her front legs high, then sticking her head out from the stall for some affectionate scratching. We conversed in our own private language. She was so engaged, unlike the many people around me who meant well but couldn't stop talking. She was just happy to have me visit her. I was delighted to have her daily company.

I believe Chicklet knew I was ill. She kept looking at me steadfastly and would lick my hands until I removed them. She brought much happiness to me during my journey and was one of the most significant relationships I had with another sentient, non-human being. She grew fast, and by the time I completed treatment she was almost fully grown and ready to compete in races. A few years later, when I was cancer-free, I went to visit her. When she saw me, she ran around fast for quite a while and kicked her hind legs up, neighing. She offered a special show, then finally came over, nodding her head up and down like she had in the past. It was a wonderful reunion like no other and I was elated! Chicklet led me to a new appreciation of the blessings of friendship, pure and simple, in dark times.

HEART RATE VARIABILITY

A courageous heart will go forth and engage with life despite confusion and fear.

A fearful heart will be hesitant and tend to hold back.

A heavy heart will make for a gloomy, unlived life.

A compassionate heart need never carry the burden of judgment.

A forgiving heart knows the art of liberation.

A loving heart awakens the spirit of possibility and engagement with others.

—John O' Donohue (2008, 104).

Without self-dependence and meaningful relationships, we can lose heart. In many cultures the word for mind also includes the heart, the two intimately related. In Western culture, the prevailing belief is that everything, even during sleep, is solely regulated by the brain. But the brain doesn't act alone; brain-like cells are located within the heart, and the brain and heart are connected through a common network. Neuro-cardiology has discovered that there is two-way communication between the brain and the heart, influencing other functions in the body and mind (Church, 2014). We know that in utero the heart is the first structured mass of tissue to form, about six weeks after conception, and it is the pulse of the first heartbeat that sets the development of all other organs in motion.

We can think of the heart as a place of arrival and departure, the blood moving in and out, being cleansed in the process. It is possible to be declared brain-dead, even while the heart keeps beating and pumping blood. The heart is the first and last organ to function within the lifespan of a human being. In many religious and spiritual traditions, the heart is the central and focal point for experiencing loving-kindness and devotion. When our hearts are open, we are receptive to other people's feelings and needs; we welcome this most powerful, healing amity, and love flows freely.

Heart rate variability shows the cyclic peaks and dips between each heartbeat. When we are stressed out and emotionally activated by an internal or external stimulus, the variance from it demonstrates pronounced high and low spikes. The differences from one heartbeat to the next can be disruptive to the natural functioning of the heart. Calming the mind with breath work and meditation brings heart coherence and regulates the heart back into its own natural rhythm and functioning. This leads to greater resilience and limits the refractory period resulting from destructive emotions, reducing it to a few hours. Without these interventions, some people remain depressed for years. If the refractory period is long, the heart rate variability is more unsettled, which takes a toll and adds injury to the body, heart, and mind. Part of becoming self-reliant is learning techniques to boost the immune system and prevent depleting it with additional stressors.

Most life stressors, such as losing a job, going through a divorce, or having close friends or family members move far away, are upsetting in the short run but usually dealt with over the course of months or years. Most people recover. Having uninvited rogue cells roaming around in one's body is ultra-stressful, and the most dangerous aspect is not having a positive guarantee of recovery. Knowing that the cancer developed over an extended period of time, without our awareness, increases our fear.

Caregivers also experience stress and burnout. If we habitually avoid releasing tension in our bodies and minds, we will eventually snap and break down. A considerable number of attendees in stress reduction classes are teachers, nurses, physicians, police officers, and other service personnel who care tremendously about others and believe in their vocations. However, not many practice self-care regularly. As the daily stuff of life takes over, people who have put off resourcing themselves crash from exhaustion. An imbalance between doing and being will bring any body to its knees.

Becky was a social worker who was very involved in the LGBT community and specialized in providing therapy and other services for cancer and AIDS patients within the LGBT population. She saw up to a dozen patients every day except for Sundays, which she spent with her wife. After thirty years of providing therapy, she found out that she had a rare type of blood cancer. She didn't seem to worry and continued to work her regular schedule for several months, until she collapsed.

She was taken to a local community hospital and was there for two weeks, in pain, undergoing many blood transfusions, and not improving. She was finally transferred to Mass General, in Boston, where she died three days later with her partner next to her. Mostly comatose, Becky didn't recognize her wife at the end. She did wake up for a few minutes, stared at her partner, speechless, never connecting. Then she fell unconscious again and, shortly after, let go of her final breath.

Becky's hard work, generosity, dedication, and kindness in supporting so many people through their pain and suffering didn't reward her during her final days. Maybe she'd needed to pace herself more and balance her working life with some personal interests. We cannot know for sure if that would have spared her from cancer, but providing too much care for others and neglecting balance in one's own life doesn't earn anyone any honor medals.

Her partner, unable to deal with the loss, committed suicide twenty-four hours before the funeral. They were buried together, which was a small consolation for the LGBT community but left its members behind in shock, with renewed anger at any kind of cancer or other terminal illness.

I have noticed a striking increase in people being diagnosed with active cancer cells shortly after they retire, maybe having waited too long, or not having had the means, to withdraw from regular employment earlier. Becky's way of managing illness is not uncommon with people working in the service field. I have also seen this in people who don't know when to quit when they are at the height of their careers or endeavors, people who don't release the continual stress in their lives, and those who are not involved in a community that fosters other interests and passions besides work.

This was the case for me too. I had to learn not to push the limits in such a way that my body could not maintain homeostasis. For a while, I had neglected to create balance between my world of accomplishments and the contemplative world of reflection and stillness. Consequently, I became confused and was suspended in a liminal world for a while.

RECOGNIZING OBSTACLES IN CAREGIVING

Let's explore some obstacles and trouble spots in caregiving, because good intentions in and of themselves don't necessarily meet the needs of those who receive the care. There are many unwholesome ways to be with someone who is ill or possibly dying, particularly when awareness is lacking or one's personal agenda supersedes the care of another. Below are five forms of dysfunctional caregiving practices.

OMNISCIENCE

I remember when I started working in a hospital and had to shadow a chaplain. In our first visit together, the chaplain entered the room of a patient who was dying from late-stage cancer. He said, "May God bless you and heal you." This happened to be a direct invasion of her space. He had not introduced us or checked her chart. She didn't give us permission to stay in the room. She was agnostic and took issue with the remark. I was very upset about his lack of sensitivity and his possible need to impress me. I reported the behavior to my supervisor who felt my concern was warranted. Our duty was not to do missionary work but to explore the patient's needs and basic concerns. Ideally, professional caregivers practice "not knowing" as a way of being, allowing the truth of each situation to emerge without having to necessarily direct it.

CONTROLLING BEHAVIOR AND IMPATIENCE

With cancer cells roaming around their bodies, patients must learn to let go of so much and enter new territories. But often a family member, insensitive to the patient's needs, will boss other family members around. They claim to know what is best, without asking in the moment what would ultimately serve the person lying there, conscious and awake. Family issues that have not been resolved will surface between family members and be a distraction from the basic needs of the patient, who has become infantilized.

Patients need caregivers to let them do what they want for as long as they can. There is no need to take over another person's life as they are losing it. Trust the sick individual's inherent wisdom and avoid the quasi-heroic urge to fix everything. Acts of heroism, sacrificing for the benefit of recognition, are irrelevant. Give up control, take a rest, and make room in your life so you can step back and gain perspective on ways to be present.

A Swiss patient with a stage III blood cancer went skiing between bouts of chemo. Her oncologist didn't like the idea. Nobody could stop her, and she was happiest skiing down the majestic mountains of Montana and Idaho until a few days before she died.

Another patient I knew, whose brother was dying of colon cancer, sent me an email saying that his brother was really stubborn and didn't want to let go and die. This was a rather strange comment from him, given that he'd had three metastases himself in the last fourteen years, and resolved to live longer than anyone else in the group.

An intolerance of pain, fear, or weariness can lead us into precarious territory, irrespective of interventions or eventualities. The course of illness or death has its own timing. Miracles happen at every step of the way, even when suffering is acute. Learn to be with what is.

INTERFERENCE

Encroaching in a fundamental way is another pitfall. Often caregivers talk too much, give unsolicited advice, try to entertain, or divert the conversation for their own benefit. Do not interrupt or direct the course of someone else's life according to your standards.

Some caregivers exhibit a loose sense of boundaries. Let's be aware of our intentions and motivation. We have to discern when we can be of service and ask what needs to be done. We let kindness and unconditional love guide us in how to be present.

SELF-SERVING AGENDAS

Occasionally, care partners want gratitude and reassurance. It is important to remember the aphorism "Don't expect applause." We surrender our hunger for praise and acknowledgment. We show up without seeking rewards or spiritual inflation. We do not know what is spiritually best for another person. Let's consider impermanence and stay open to what unfolds. Presence and unconditional love are aspects of being spiritual that bring us humility in the face of any illness.

EMPATHIC DISTRESS

Empathy with a patient can engender a harmful distortion. Empathic distress means that someone is associating with the suffering, taking it in, not able to release it, overwhelmed by the ordeal. We let go of being attached to the person in need. Staying open to discomfort, we use it as an opportunity to see our expectations, fears, and ideas. Another's suffering can be a catalyst for compassionate care.

Most importantly, we give up the notion of a good death! Each death is unique. There are a great many fantasies about a good death. Do not put any pressure on the dying person. Instead, relax and let go of expectations. People leave at their own pace. I have noticed patients in the hospital die while their loved ones step out to grab a bite or break up their visit. Preparing for death before one gets sick is certainly beneficial. No one knows how they will fare when the moment arrives. It is important to build emotional muscles and learn to gain resolve.

CULTIVATING LOVING-KINDNESS AND COMPASSION

Between ideas of right and wrong, there is a place. I'll meet you there.

—Rumi

Traditional Judeo-Christian culture is based on the basic premise that we are born deficient, fractured sinners. This odd birthmark makes for a difficult start in life. Our innate goodness is buried deep under the dogma that we are flawed and therefore in dire need of redemption.

It is hardly possible to love others if we don't love ourselves. I don't mean a narcissistic love based on a constant need to be acknowledged or admired. I mean the recognition that we need to appreciate ourselves for who we are in every moment of our existence. Inevitably, we fall down, and then we get up and improve our lot. When we take detours from our path, we find a way back to the road leading home.

Self-compassion is an inner ally that leads to a reduction of negative mind states, shame, and anxiety. It has a soft, grandmotherly quality, as well as a fierce, tough love aspect that honors our need for protection. We are not victims who dwell in blame displacement or self-indulgence. Instead, sensing our common humanity, we have caring concern for our bodies, minds, and spirits. Self-compassion is linked to satisfaction, gratitude, contentment, and the immune system. It lessens the fear of failure, which is exhausting, and gives us instead resources to support others.

Vested in altruistic behavior and the greater common good, we are human, tender, vulnerable, and curious. We are one of the few mammals that walk upright with our bellies and hearts exposed. It is not selfish to care for ourselves. When we love ourselves, with our whole repertoire of strengths and liabilities, we can make changes along the way to better ourselves. We cultivate and develop altruism, a motivational state that improves the welfare of others and champions freedom and wisdom. Support groups allow members to develop loving-kindness for themselves and each other in the midst of struggles, providing changes in their physical, emotional, and cognitive worlds that are affected by chemo brain.

A few years ago, several women who attended one of the groups got together and had a party for another member who was about to have a radical mastectomy. Prior to the surgery, clay breasts were cast from the woman's own. At the party, members decorated bras with great imagination, which made all the women smile, laugh, and cry. It is never easy to give up body parts, no matter how damaged they are. Shortly thereafter, a lingerie shop owner who had formerly had breast cancer, started a yearly, wild bra-decorating show that has been duplicated throughout the country to raise funds.

Support groups give participants a safe container for finding purpose, opening their hearts, connecting with their breath, and welcoming the paradoxical, unexpected, and inconceivable. Members show little hesitancy to go deep, exploring and sharing tenderness, strengths, commonalities, woes, and their very distinct approaches to intimacy and comfort, if only for a few cherished moments. Frequently, members bond enough to get together outside of the group setting, share rides to and from appointments, and connect around common interests.

Kelly, a former ballet dancer with Martha Graham's company, reluctantly came to one of the cancer support groups, because her best friend ordered her to join. She was a loner and because her ovarian cancer was at stage IV, she didn't have much hope. Her timing was not propitious, as a couple of members were in the process of dying, looking haggard, wearing barely any flesh on their bones, covering their heads with wigs and hats, and suffering intense discomfort. The ballerina had lived as a recluse for years, due to an injury from a car accident that shortened her dancing career. She was very poor by any standard. She'd refused to undergo any treatment. At the end of the first meeting, she promised that she would think about joining the group. When she came back two weeks later, another member offered to drive her to Mass General Hospital for chemo treatments.

Today, after ten years, a trip to Greece, studying the Greek language and history, two clinical trials, a liver ablation, and many other invasive treatments, she is on maintenance chemotherapy. There are no more magic concoctions available at this juncture. She turned eighty, had an amazing, intense journey and even developed a platonic love affair with her mensch of an oncologist. She attends the group on a regular basis, is included and appreciated, and gives and receives much-needed love to and from the other group members.

Empathy, altruism, and loving-kindness require courage. When we experience overwhelming fear and insecurity, it is difficult to have empathy and feel another person's suffering from within. Compassion is wanting someone's suffering to be diminished, or removed, with tenderness from the heart. The first element of compassion is empathy, feeling suffering for another being. If we stop here, we risk burnout and become unable to cultivate productive social behavior.

Once we resource ourselves, we can reappraise negative situations from a healthier perspective. Compassion includes the deep resolve to engage in an intelligent response, making contact with our own vulnerabilities and tender hearts. It is an active process which requires a template for immediate, mediated presence.

When ill, we need to love ourselves just the way we are. There is no need to look for reasons to torture ourselves with blame, criticism, and guilt. Nor must care partners become bleeding hearts, compelled to save others. When not grounded in reality, a tendency to place the needs of others above one's own is dangerous and unsustainable. Cultivating compassion is a gradual process and not a romantic notion or idealized state. Neither is it relegated to idle good wishes or pity.

In 2004, I met a trauma resiliency expert who was working with NGOs after a tsunami hit Indonesia, providing services to indigenous people. On her way to start a busy day helping others, she ran into a tall, elderly woman standing by the beach with a distant look in her eyes, her body barely clothed. The counselor asked how she could help her. The elder said, "If you came here to help me, don't bother. If you came here to share your liberation with mine, we may walk together." This was an earth-shattering response from a person stripped of everything, who was not being swept away by terrible circumstances and losses. We never know how resilient people will be or who will show up, destitute or prospering, with fierceness and tenderness in the midst of the most unimaginable circumstances.

We can attend to ourselves and the space where another resides so that they might open up and be assured that they will not be abandoned. Otherwise, fear doesn't allow any room for the compassion required to meet someone else's needs.

When I was on call at a local hospital, the nurses would often ask me to deal with an eighty-five-year-old woman who had no family. Her only friend was her pastor. She needed lots of attention, and the short-staffed night shift nurses didn't have spare time to spend with her. The frail, petite, terminally ill woman was often distressed and wanted to share her woes with someone. After many calls from the nurses' station requesting my intervention, I decided I would just sit or lie next to her in the tiny medical bed, holding her hand. No words were needed. She quieted down and breathed slower. I matched my breath with hers and remained silent. From then on, she would most times fall asleep instantly.

I would leave quietly, walking by the nurses' station to give a thumbs-up, letting them know that she was resting comfortably. I did this without mentioning the magic of touch, which was against hospital rules. Though patient protections and hospital liabilities are legitimate and indispensable, sometimes we are called upon to act outside of linear thinking and unproductive, impersonal standards in order to effectively serve the patient and healthcare providers. Of course, this prompted more calls from the nurses for other patients disturbing the order of their unit. It's clear to me that in our later years we become more childlike again, appreciating soothing physical contact more often than words that might sound hollow. When one has been lying in bed for many days and nights due to illness, one can detect within seconds whether another person stepping in the room is ill at ease. A slight touch and often deep silence will give the patient some space to befriend their oceanic exhaustion.

The more we open ourselves to compassion, the more we will be tested. By uncoupling our habitual narratives, we realize that few things separate us from other sentient beings except our judgments and our skin. We can practice non-referential compassion, having no preferences and biases for a "special tribe" or exclusive friendships. Non-referential compassion implies that we don't privilege people we like over those we dislike; we don't dismiss anyone. Having compassion for oneself or someone else is an antidote to attachment, cruelty, jealousy, envy, and ignorance. It is a path to reconnection with others.

Goleman and Davidson (2017) explain that loving-kindness and compassion meditation practices, over the long term, are a direct way to move beyond one's concerns and obsessions. There is a practice called Lojong, or Tonglen, that provides a path to liberation from afflictive mental states, transforming suffering into freedom. The body and mind undergo ceaseless transformations even though we wish for qualities of permanence and autonomy. Our bodies are temporary assemblages of flesh and bones; our personal histories are but a memory of what is no more; and our identities change constantly.

This means we are essentially a dynamic stream of experiences interrupted by the need for ego revelations, which are simply threads of narrow mental space and, at times, a self-imposed prison. When we cultivate altruistic love and compassion, rumination and self-absorption lessen. Once we start to serve in capacities to generate connection, we gain strength and satisfaction, and the world brightens. Moving beyond the personal self, we become benefactors: happiness manifests from within, in the service of others.

TONGLEN MEDITATION: THE PRACTICE OF TAKING AND GIVING

Tonglen is one of the most cherished Buddhist practices. The enactment of compassion is the taking component, and the enactment of loving-kindness is the giving component. This practice may alleviate the suffering of others, but the true criterion of success is the attenuation of our own self-centeredness and the growth of love and compassion in our own hearts. The real litmus test for our practice is to recognize how we deal with harmful people.

Bring to mind as vividly as possible your mother, father, sibling, or child, whom you care about deeply. In other words, one of the beings who is most precious in your life. Perhaps the cause of their suffering is physical, psychological, social, or environmental. For a moment, empathetically embrace their suffering, and in your mind's eye, bring forth the wish: "May they be relieved of their burden."

Whatever the burden or affliction of your loved one, imagine taking it in as a black cloud. Draw and funnel it into your heart so that the person is relieved. As soon as this dark cloud enters your heart, imagine and visualize it as an orb of darkness that becomes extinguished.

Emanate a wellspring of brilliant, radiant white light of joy and virtue from your heart, reaching the person, and you may say, "All that is good in my life, my good health, my happiness, my good virtues of the past, present and future, I offer you. May your greatest yearnings for well-being and deepest aspirations in life be fulfilled."

There is no need to worry that the suffering will overwhelm you or that the luminosity of your heart, flowing unceasingly, will be depleted. Its source is inexhaustible. Now, take a couple of deep breaths and rest for a while.

The next steps repeat the process, focusing on the suffering of those who are progressively more removed from us:

- a friend
- an acquaintance
- someone you dislike or even despise
- and all sentient beings in the world

Finally, draw your awareness into your own body, and imagine the radiant, luminous white light of virtue and joy emanating from your heart and suffusing your body. Realize that the light cannot be contained, with its rays emitting from every pore of your body in all directions.

Complete your practice with a dedication: "By the merit of this practice, may every sentient being gain liberation from suffering and the sources of suffering. May the deepest yearning of each be fulfilled."

For a couple of minutes, rest with the good intention of being free of any obscurations, and be at ease.

LIVING BEYOND COPING

The purpose of life is a life of purpose.

—Robert Byrne

Purpose is vital for our psychological and emotional well-being, particularly when we are limited by illness. It is an opportunity for us to orient ourselves based on our values and intentions. It is a way to stay connected to our experiences, regardless of whether we are rewarded by them or not. Sometimes, disappointment gives us an impetus to strive harder.

This was the case for Drora, who was diagnosed with stage IV lung cancer even though she had never smoked in her life. She travels all over the country and abroad to raise awareness and money for people with her diagnosis. There is much prejudice against lung cancer patients due to a pervasive assumption that lung cancer is just a smoker's disease. This stigma obstructs funding for this type of cancer. Drora is remarkable because her rogue cells metastasized in her brain, and yet three brain surgeries later she is still fighting the stigma. Her fierce motivation keeps her alive.

Drora was inspired to take action from a place of empathy. The etymology of "empathy" comes, in part, from the German word *Einfühlung*, which refers to the ability to sense from within what another person is feeling. Empathy can arise when we have feelings for a person with whom we enter into resonance. True empathic concern consists of becoming aware of another's needs and meeting them through listening and beneficial strategies that affirm and support their wishes. It doesn't involve pity, which is extremely condescending.

Loving-kindness and compassion do wonders. Healing is accelerated by caring for oneself and others.

FOCUSING ON INTENTION NOT OUTCOME

When you help, you see life as weak. When you fix, you see life as broken. When you serve, you see life as whole.

—Rachel Naomi Remen, MD

A classic reaction to any unexpected event is blame displacement. Casting blame outward prevents us from looking inward for the support of our own resources and strength. Adopting a victim's stance is a dead-end road. We always have options to change and improve the quality of our lives. There are many victims in the world blaming others for their "stuckness" and looking for rescuers to do their work. They replicate the lives of rogue cells on a collective and political level. The immune system can only grow and become stronger when we choose to broaden our outlook and responses. This intention gives us an impetus to be less unconscious. The Tibetan cattle herders have a saying, "In order to better manage cattle, one has to give them a greater pasture." In my experience, more spaciousness works well for most of us, lessening control and aggression. When safety isn't the most urgent thing in our lives, our capacity for getting on with, and embracing, aliveness increases. Altruistic intentions without a neurotic concern for positive rewards open up vast fields of kindness.

Many of the people I have walked with over the years had benefactors and were part of a lineage of benefactors themselves, receiving and giving unconditional love. Even when sick they demonstrated empathy, loving-kindness, and compassion, becoming benefactors rather than a burden to family, friends, and strangers. Benefactors tend to live longer than those who drown in the downward spiral of the deep well of sorrow and depression.

I remember one group member being asked by her friends what would be of support to her. She asked her church members to send her cards, uplifting or funny ones, asking for their permission to respond and express her anger. She replied with words about cancer cells that cannot be put in print here. Unshackling her feelings was perfect relief for her. Her friends obliged and supported her fully in that manner.

Sally, a member of an ovarian cancer support group, decided to make stars out of cloth and fill them with dry grains. She gave them to people so they could remember that they are stars, even while sick. She wanted to change her outlook and predicament by doing something that would benefit others. She lived for eleven years beyond her prognosis and made over seventeen thousand stars, giving them to people affected by cancer. She regularly mailed me a box filled with them. They fit in the palm of one's hand and provide a soft, malleable squeeze of comfort. Pure tenderness! I carry several in my briefcase and give them out to new support group members. She is a shining star to me and very much alive in many people's minds and hearts, even though she left us recently. I went to her memorial, where hundreds gathered to honor her, in awe of her spirit living among us.

DROPPING INTO PRESENCE

I have learned that people will forget what you said, people will forget what you did, but people will never forget how you made them feel.

—Maya Angelou

Presence is the quality of being-through-listening, resonating with others, bearing witness, respecting one's inner space, getting out of one's way, and letting go of obsessive inner chatter. Often, presence is communicated non-verbally, and others can sense and feel this quality of being without fear. Silent presence creates intimacy and connection so that people can release unsettled emotional material without interruption or commentary. This special way of being allows us to be emotionally available and accessible in a way that clarifies intention and invites connection. Being present is also an invitation to take a vulnerable plunge into the unknown.

Support groups foster a sense of inclusivity in order for members to maintain sanity during severe illness. As long as the leader and participants notice strong biases, groupthink, and prejudices about survival strategies or emotional resonance components that get in the way, the group fosters a deep sense of belonging, which replaces the loss of one's old notion of identity and autonomy. Despair, loneliness, and shortsightedness recede in the face of courage and strength. Groups are a platform for caring, sharing special needs, and discussing common afflictions. They are a hub where people can find relief, be seen, and are permitted to drop their long-worn masks. When we are grounded and have a sense of resonance with others, there is a larger sense of spaciousness and expansion in our connections.

WAY OF COUNCIL

The following exercise assists us in being transparent in a group, family, community, or healthcare setting. This model is superb for gaining transparency, interacting with others to develop listening skills, and investing in a responsible dialogue, not a debate. Whenever someone wants to speak in a group setting, they hold a talking piece which can be any object one chooses to hold in one's hand. This allows the speaker to talk freely without being interrupted or receiving feedback, advice, or suggestions. When the speaker is done, the talking piece is given to the next person who wishes to speak.

There are several levels to the Way of Council (Zimmerman and Coyle 1996), but the basic model has five principal guidelines:

1. Speak from the heart and reveal what is meaningful in the moment

2. Be concise, go to essence

3. Be spontaneous

4. Listen from the heart

5. Honor confidentiality

This is a great vehicle for sharing meaning in the present moment and being heard and seen without unnecessary commentaries. Often, remarkable insights arise because there are no interruptions or anyone finishing the speaker's sentences. There is an organic unfolding of revelations that surface because participants have the time to pause and unearth aspects of themselves that otherwise wouldn't emerge. There is also time to choose precise language to frame ideas and intentions. It allows people to witness the genuine, common human traits of trust, patience, respect, and compassion. It fosters sincere interest in relating with one another, dropping into our basic goodness, shared suffering, joy, and gifts.

BECOMING RESILIENT

One can only face in others what one can face in oneself.

—James Baldwin

It is difficult to be resilient given all the challenges patients or caregivers face around illness. Resilience is the ability to face and handle challenges—big ones, ostensibly insurmountable ones. We can move beyond surprises, disappointments, betrayals, and paradoxes. The Latin word *paradoxum* means that something is seemingly contradictory, but true in fact; in other words, it is an insult to our rational mind. We can either recover quickly from adversity or become crippled by it. Why do some of us cave in when encountering barriers in life? Why do some of us concede to and espouse whatever life throws at us?

The capacity to bounce back from an upsetting event, to integrate it and then move on, is an innate triumph. In its most elemental form, this is called coping. As I have mentioned before, we can move from post-traumatic stress to posttraumatic growth. The left prefrontal cortex lights up during an MRI when resilience increases, while the right side of the prefrontal cortex is more active, sending inhibitory signals to the amygdala, instructing it to calm down. The mind relaxes the brain when we activate resilience because it grows new connections, pathways, and circuits, which reinforce new attitudes in our mental and emotional world (Goleman and Davidson 2017).

We can use cognitive reappraisal of distressing events to reframe adversity in such a way that it is no longer perceived as extreme. Rather than pathologizing, we can view an event as a mistake or inadequacy and improve the efficacy of our thoughts. Cultivating empathy for oneself is a great antidote for dis-regulation and temporary discomfort. Always remember your basic goodness, your inner nobility, and emulate people who function at optimal levels, being the best versions of themselves.

Look at the following list of basic suggestions to cultivate resilience. Pick one or two that are most difficult to relate to and explore what barriers stand in the way of adopting them.

• Develop a core set of beliefs that nothing or nobody can shake.

• Try to find meaning in whatever stressful phenomena have surfaced in your life.

• Maintain a wholesome vision and focus on what brings aliveness and vividness.

• Take cues from and emulate beings who are resilient, grounded, and authentic.

• Don't run from things that scare you; face them.

• Reach out for support when things go haywire.

• Learn new things as often as you can.

• Find an exercise regimen to follow every other day and stick to it.

• Don't beat yourself up or dwell on the past.

• Be aware of what makes you uniquely strong and special, and own it.

• Have faith in something larger than yourself.

• Join a community of support.

While some of these suggestions seem unreachable, consider maybe one of them. Look at the upside of what the change might bring, not just the downside. Maybe spend five minutes contemplating the meaning behind the words. They ask you to enter a greater field of awareness and there is nothing to lose. You do not have to come up with immediate answers. Ask someone in your support group how they might overcome deficiencies about meeting their goals for an improved attitude.

BUILDING A COMMUNITY OF SUPPORT

When your eyes are tired
the whole world is tired also.

. . . .

You must learn one thing.
The world was made to be free in.

Give up all the other worlds
except the one to which you belong.

Sometimes it takes darkness and the sweet
confinement of your aloneness
to learn

anything or anyone
that doesn't bring you alive

is too small for you.
(David Whyte, "Sweet Darkness" 1997)

There are many communities available for people with cancer. Some raise money, organize walks, five- or ten-mile races, dances, and other related events. Many add activities, such as painting, writing, knitting, and drumming classes. Others focus on physical exercise, such as kayaking, dancing, or yoga, and some participate in the Live Strong program. All groups are important for bonding, sharing commonalities and resources, opening up to the many strong emotions that surface, learning to name them and let them dissipate.

There are many important practical issues for patients to deal with: exploring financial considerations, getting free transportation or meals, formulating a will, evaluating what type of funeral services are required, and other issues that need to be addressed and resolved. Questions rise to the surface about how do to deal with chemo brain and neuropathy, whether or not to utilize CBD with THC or wear a wig, who to share the circumstances of the illness with and when, and so many other details.

"The fellowship of those who bear the mark of pain," as my childhood hero Dr. Albert Schweitzer called it, is a safe container in which attendees find ways to talk about their deepest emotions, hidden secrets, and uncommon experiences, without having to worry about being judged or shamed. Members realize that they have been visiting the underworld, facing their demons several times over, yet few whine. Common concerns need to be addressed and there are individual ways to handle them efficiently. Some people are running out of treatment options and getting ready for hospice care as new people join the group. This can be intimidating for new members. However, the experience of connectedness to a greater whole supports them in exploring unfamiliar emotional depths. They can see that other members have gained resilience, peace of mind, and that most are not afraid to die. Much fear is rooted in a reluctant dependence on others for basic needs: toileting and intimate hygiene, hair washing (if any remains), or even just mobility.

Fear of recurrence often lurks in the back of someone's mind whose body was invaded by rogue cells. We know the anticipation of recurrence is an irrational thought, and yet it does manifest. For many, the thought of having to go through another chemo or radiation journey pops up every so often, sometimes even decades after having been discharged by the oncologist. One rarely challenges or contests this kind of rejection! Rather, we welcome the dismissal, perhaps with some hesitation or a moment of disbelief. It takes time to sink in, and effort to begin another chapter in life. Many patients, even years later, as they continue to participate in their group, will have rare moments of anticipatory anxiety as they meet new participants who are very sick. They never again want to be physically weak, emotionally distraught, or at the start of another cancer journey. The anxiety does not usually last long, as experienced patients know the mind can go there very easily.

In the group, attendees transform their deep humiliation and loneliness, embrace their new compulsory identity, and earn a well-deserved membership from a community of those who are mindful and strive to be alive as best they can. Many of the emerging concerns discussed in each group have to do with family, friends, and coworkers who don't know what to say or how to relate. Sometimes they ask how they can help. Dr. Naomi Rachel Remen (2000) emphasizes service as a preferred alternative to help. I invite anyone who cares about an ailing person to ask them how they can best be served, a simple question that will reach out to them with an expression of heartfelt concern and support. In order to serve anyone who is in need, or experiencing pain, and honor their deepest essence, we let go of our selfish wishes and agendas and keep asking questions.

The Mountain Meditation focuses on a symbol of strength that is a great metaphor for standing steadfast while weathering changes and surprises. Mountains contain a multitude of minerals, plants, and animals. These might not be easily visible, but the mountain is composed of them just like we are composed of our inner resources and potential.

MOUNTAIN MEDITATION

Let the body and mind settle in their natural functioning. Breathing normally, not too tight, not too loose, just be aware of the breath that carries you through life. Breathing in, fill the abdomen and lungs. Breathing out, empty and release all tensions and contractions.

Consider being a mountain, sitting tall and firm. Bring to mind a mountain that you have seen. Walk up to the summit and hold it in your mind's eye. The base is rooted, large, unmoving, perfectly stable. So is your body, majestic in its powerful, natural presence and girth.

Notice the points of contact where your body meets the chair, cushion, or floor. You don't need to know where one ends or begins; the base is an extension of yourself. Your arms are like the slopes of the mountain, a home and refuge for many living things.

The spine is erect and majestic, soaring upward like the mountain's peak. Your head is the lofty summit, floating above the clouds, under the vast sky.

Sit in silence, mountain-like, unmoved by the changing of seasons, day to night, pleasant and turbulent weather patterns, gusty winds, or smooth breezes.

The mountain is always anchored, grounded, and stable. Your mind might rage like a storm, but the body rests steadfast, and you are able to let the elements pass by.

Sensing the mountain reminds you of your innate strength and beauty, your basic goodness, your stability and dignity. You witness the continuous passage of thoughts, sensations, and feelings.

You are serene, experiencing ease and peace in your whole being.

Equanimity

Two monks were talking amongst themselves outside the temple. One said to the other monk, "The flag is moving." The other said, "The wind is moving." The teacher who was sitting nearby said, "Not the flag, not the wind, dear monks; the mind is moving."

—The Platform Sutra of the 6th Patriarch Hui Neng,

Chan Buddhist scripture

Equanimity is like the bright moon reflecting the light of the sun in the dark-blue night sky. The cooler quality of the moon doesn't represent any lack of caring. Equanimity means tolerance, impartiality, letting go, not choosing one thing over another. It doesn't mean being in a state of complete balance between extremes, nor is it indifference. It is the state of accepting things inclusively, seeing the full picture, and looking at circumstances from all angles. When we are not in opposition to anything, we neither make things worse, nor repress or suppress anything, nor do we judge the situation at hand. We inquire and discern what is beneficial when there is suffering in ourselves or someone else. When we are grateful, we have and cause no fear and are rewarded with ample freedom.

Before I became intimately acquainted with the disease myself, I had a colleague who had pancreatic cancer. We often worked together on special health programs and projects. When I went to visit him at the hospital, I was frightened, not sure what to say or how to behave. I was actually sweating, going up in the elevator. When I entered the room, he was sitting on his medical bed, propped up against pillows. He was a large man of African descent, but the color of his skin was yellowish now. Ill at ease, I kept talking about business, until he finally stopped me and said, "Please sit down next to me. Pierre, you don't have to say anything or be uncomfortable. I am ok. Work is over for me. I am very pleased that you came. It tends to be lonely here, and I appreciate you visiting me. It is a great gift. Thank you."

I was relieved, and I received the best lesson ever about presence. After a half hour or so, we said our goodbyes and hugged. He died a week later. I went to the cathedral of the Abyssinian Baptist Church, in Harlem, for his memorial. I cried a lot while the spectacular choir sang, and Reverend Dr. Calvin Butts and many others spoke of my friend's astounding life. Afterward, I walked about thirty blocks through Harlem, a part of New York unfamiliar to me, in a three-piece suit, looking for a cab. I wasn't successful in hailing one, but the stroll was refreshing, and it gave me an occasion to process my colleague's beautiful legacy. My friend was at peace, and his grace and serenity channeled through me, leaving a lifelong impression. He had found the equanimity that I would later need to cultivate for myself, during my own journey with cancer.

KEEPING THE MIND BIG AND SPACIOUS

When we consider that the world of experience exists only in relation to the mind that perceives it, it becomes easier to understand its nature. In the Dhammapada, Buddha defined our experiences by saying, "All phenomena are preceded by the mind, issued forth from the mind, and consist of the mind" (Wallace 2009, 177). This is one of the most convincing explanations of the workings of the mind, because while the body is dear to us, and we are able to express ourselves with our voices, the mind holds the most important place.

Some neuroscientists believe that mental processes originate in the brain, yet they are not the same as neural bases, bear no physical qualities, and cannot be objectively measured. According to B. Alan Wallace (2009, 25), this "undermines the value of introspection, and implicitly supports the assumption that mental processes are really nothing more than brain processes viewed from a subjective perspective. The implication is that brain processes are real, but mental processes are illusory". This is obviously not the case, even though consciousness is invisible to our physical and objective means of observation. Paying attention to the mind supports us in seeing mental images, thoughts, and different forms of consciousness that can only be expressed by first-person experience. I am drawn to Siegel's definition of the multi- faceted mind as "an embodied and relational, emergent self-organizing process that regulates energy and information flow" (2017, 62). This explanation of the mind regulating energy supports the notion that with equanimity we choose to hold a more wholesome and broad view. According to Siegel (2017, 69-70), the "science of the mind" explores a series of "subjective, mental experiences" that have a natural drive and link differentiated parts into a coherent whole; this integration underlies health, resilience, and well-being.

Let's look at the relationship between the brain and the mind. What are their specific and distinct functions? How do the mind, brain, and consciousness differ or relate to each other? The mind, defined as consciousness, has no location in the body. The brain is matter, comprised of atoms and molecules from the elements: earth, water, fire, air, and space. Matter can be measured, qualified, and quantified. Mind, compared with the brain, is unconditioned, intangible, has no color or shape, is boundless and beyond categories. Mind experiences unconditional love. It is awareness: the realization of the relationship we have with any phenomena we direct our attention to. Together, synchronized but each maintaining its own integrity, the brain and the mind are concerned with the nature of being, the human condition, and making peace with the world we inhabit. They must coexist and co-create in order to achieve health and harmony.

When the mind becomes agitated and turbulent, strong emotions arise and constrict the ego. Mindfulness practices allow us to regulate these disturbing emotions and see the inclusive picture and the choices available. The Tibetan Buddhist term for ego means a "magical display," because it is invested in taking positions that have little to do with what goes on in the moment. When we discover the nature of mind, we are able to realize that *everything* is mind; everything rises, moves, changes, and returns to the manifestation of the "natural state" of the mind, which is spacious and free.

The mind can be a friend or foe. Often, we become slaves to our thoughts, chasing after them as if they were the experience itself, completely losing sight of the fact that a thought is only a manifestation of the nature of the mind. We don't want our minds to control us. We can be in charge by being aware and paying attention to the relationship we have with any object of attention. When thoughts arise, we see them for what they are, appearances of the mind, empty in and of themselves. They don't have that much power or influence over us unless we assign it to them.

There was once a samurai who consulted a Buddhist priest with regard to understanding heaven and hell. He said to the teacher, "Explain to me what heaven and hell is. If you cannot answer I will cut your head off with my sword!" The priest said, "You are an idiot and won't understand the difference between the two." At that moment, the samurai drew his sword. The priest said, "That is hell." The samurai sheathed his sword back into the scabbard. The priest said, "That is heaven!" The samurai bowed to the priest and left. This is a perfect example, explaining how mind and action are synchronized in order for equanimity to surface.

Each time we become aware of an object, event, or thought, consciousness presents us with an appearance, which is its interpretation of the object, event, or thought. Appearances are impermanent, and anything brought into existence by the mind is dependent upon a conceptual designation. Consciousness works directly with what appears in any experience, and it has a tendency to build up a model, or construct, of something that exists beyond mere appearances. Meditation practices help us suspend the habit of continually ascribing some concrete existence to everything we experience. Instead, we let sensations, feelings, and thoughts, rise, dissipate, and rest in quiescence. We observe the movements of the mind, just like when we watch the waves coming to shore and receding. The movements of the mind keep appearing and dissipating over and over. Quiescence provides a pause much like the one between any inhalation and exhalation, maybe lasting longer and longer as we drop into the practice and the ground of being. Awareness is always present, but because we are caught up in doing, we rarely notice.

Meditation becomes the art of listening, the space in which thoughts occur. Awareness and quiet are the most intimate characteristics of consciousness. The sacred and timeless are present in the background of every experience and are not battling with the mind.

SAVORING GRACE

Many times a day I realize how much my own outer and inner life is built upon the labors of my fellow men, both living and dead, and how earnestly I must exert myself in order to give in return as much as I have received.

—Albert Einstein

It is important to check out what our aspirations are, what direction we want to go about setting the compass of our hearts to, and give ourselves room to experience bodily sensations and emotions. The brain is wired in a way that is not necessarily conducive to awareness and expressions of gratitude. Unpleasant experiences are stored in our long-term memory, but pleasant experiences go into short-term memory and linger only briefly. This explains why it is hard to let go of unsettling and inconvenient experiences. Traumatic events tend to stick around even longer, requiring intervention by a qualified clinician, who may need to employ tactics such as Eye Movement Desensitization and Reprocessing (EMDR) or the Emotional Freedom Technique (EFT) to retrieve unpleasant memories and integrate left and right brain functions. When awareness and gratitude intersect, equanimity stands a better chance to develop.

The word gratitude comes from the Latin word *gratis*, which means "thankfulness, wanting to please." Every day is a day for gratitude, and even celebrating in small ways, prevents us from becoming exhausted or killing the mind of compassion. Gratitude enables us to be part of the larger context in which our personal experiences are unfolding. It softens the heart, directs the gaze toward what is meaningful, and builds greater capacity for forgiveness. It gives us an appreciation for the interdependent nature of our existence.

Reminding ourselves of what and whom we are grateful for doesn't deny life's daily difficulties, the challenges faced by our planet, troubled financial times, uncertainties about the future, or harm caused by those close to us or more distant. Practicing gratitude lifts the veil of doom and gloom and, in place of isolation, opens a door that leads to the creation of community. We may even be grateful for those who have generated less than ideal circumstances for us, seeing that their pain and suffering are all part of a mysterious whole. When we practice gratitude and receive graciously, we also give someone else the opportunity to be generous.

Janet was a woman vicar I used to visit on the chemo infusion unit. As I knew very little about her religion, she educated and informed me about all the rituals and celebrations she attended with other women each week, even while sick. Janet was very grateful that I spent time with her as an interfaith chaplain without judging her about her spiritual path or walking away from her as so many had in her life. The fact that she didn't have to justify her beliefs, and that her faith and rituals were accepted, was a huge relief for her.

She talked energetically about her religion while chemo juices were dripping into her upper chest like a leaking faucet. Her passion was fascinating to me. I learned many aspects of her beliefs and she loved the fact that I was open to her faith-based approach to life. She was also interested in hearing about the impact of Buddhism on my life. I often stopped by when she was in the unit, enjoying her presence and animated discussions immensely, feeling grateful to know her.

Gratitude is a powerful antidote for emotional chaos, occasional despair, depression, and defeating thoughts and behaviors. It supports us in overcoming feelings of loss, scarcity, and envy. More importantly, it releases us from the fear of always wanting something more than we have.

THE NEED FOR TRANSPARENCY

You can see a lot just by watching.

—Yogi Berra

Becoming intimate with our own minds offers us ongoing insights that propel us from "stickiness" to fluidity. It is a commitment to be as honest as possible with ourselves, regardless of the progress of the Big C, exploring our shadow sides and penetrating the unconscious world of our repetitive patterns that might be convenient but not fulfilling or functional. To be transparent takes courage. To be able to shift our views, let go of solid beliefs, and bear witness to what *is* supports equanimous states within us, within the world, and for the world. Changing habitual and repetitive behaviors manifests in three primary and specific ways:

1. Being transparent to ourselves.

When we are no longer ruled by our emotions, preferences, and conditioning, we are able to shift our views and become less distracted or less likely to disperse precious energy. We don't have to make up storylines, but rather observe what is meaningful in the moment. Over time we become more proficient in letting go of unnecessary thoughts, speech, and behaviors.

2. Letting the world be transparent to us.

When we stop projecting our own ideas, opinions, and weighty judgments, we can see reality as it is—pleasant or unpleasant, exciting or boring—and not just fabricated in a certain way to make us feel better or worse. We yield and respond freely when we see things clearly and without biases.

3. Being transparent to the world

We no longer need to hide behind roles, identities, habitual patterns, personas, histories, or ego structures. We become open, undefended, meeting the world as it is, with all its beauty and cruelty.

I was sitting with a sweet, petite ninety-four-years-young lady when the chaplaincy supervisor joined us in the infusion unit. She was in charge of supervising new chaplains who were in the line of duty for the first time. I had just asked Rosalie how her day was unfolding. Mid-transfusion, she was lamenting, in pain from a late-stage renal cancer, her voice barely audible. When she found out I was a Buddhist chaplain, she wanted to learn everything about Buddhist psychology, spiritual beliefs, and cosmology. She asked many questions and thought that she might like to explore Buddhism in more depth, inviting me to come back soon. She let me know her chemotherapy schedule, making sure we could meet again to discuss the topic further. My supervisor was delighted about our session together, particularly since I was the only chaplain visiting patients at the large cancer chemotherapy and radiation center in Western Massachusetts. I was a test case for future chaplains and had to prove the need for such visits. I went to visit Rosalie weekly, until she passed away a couple of months later. She was a very curious person with an interesting history, almost a century old. I loved her kind spirit and later missed visiting her. Curiosity and an open mind are great supports and springboards for cultivating equanimity.

When adopting these three levels of transparency, we welcome everything and push away nothing. Opening up to experience, we find contentment in the midst of it all. The more transparent we are, the more authenticity and freedom will rise to the forefront and guide us in a manner that will empower us in any given situation.

COMING HOME TO ONESELF MEDITATION

One definition of the word meditation is "to come home to ourselves again and again." Sitting with a strong, equanimous back and soft front, let go of tension, loosen the belly, and breathe normally.

Be aware of the air flowing into your lungs and notice the natural pause before the air releases, slightly warmer now as it exits the body. Breathing in, we are saying "Yes!" to another moment of life with all its joy, contentment, sorrow, and loss. Breathing out, we release all of it, let go, and rest in the gap between the end of the exhalation and the next inhalation.

Coming back to simple presence is the kindest and most compassionate way to treat ourselves. We cultivate unconditional friendliness toward ourselves and our whole range of experiences.

We don't react, justify, or condemn.

We don't have to fill up the space each time there is a gap.

Each moment is a perfect teacher. We are fine when our awareness rests in the present moment and attention is focused on the mind and breath. As soon as mental events, thoughts, or feelings arise, we note them and let them go.

Little by little, over time, and with continued practice, the mind will prefer to go in the direction of peace and calm abiding.

ESPOUSING EQUANIMITY

The Great Way is not difficult for those who have no preferences.

—Jianzhi Sengcan, The Third Patriarch of Zen

Now that we have begun the radical shift of unpacking the knots we were previously blind to, we become more comfortable, dropping into a new awareness, and finding a new place to land called equanimity. Neither an eternal state of balance, nor a suspension between extremes, equanimity gives us a platform for accepting things as they are. We face uncertainty with courage and are not swept away by it. We surrender and are free from powerful reactions and pride. We discover "isness," meaning we relax the strong hold we have on things or people, and the world becomes less of an obstacle. We see things clearly, the way they are unfolding, and we let go of desired outcomes. We untangle the tangles, instead of unraveling, and we welcome one moment after the other. It's a formidable task! The benefits of eliciting, recognizing, and experiencing states of equanimity include the uncoiling of long-standing constricting patterns ruled by ignorance, delusion, and ill will. The following classic folk story illustrates this powerful notion in an unusual context.

There was a monk living at the edge of a village. One day, a young man came through the village with a work crew to rebuild a bridge for a few weeks. He befriended a young girl. They became lovers, and then he moved on when construction was finished. She soon realized that she was pregnant. When she told her parents, they asked her who the father was. She said that it was the monk at the edge of the village who was responsible for the baby. Her parents were furious and went to see the monk immediately, accusing him of getting their daughter pregnant, despite his vow of celibacy. He responded, "Is that so?" They told him that he would be responsible for bringing up the baby. He said again, "Is that so?"

They brought him the baby. He made the infant comfortable in his small hut. He subsequently took off his robes and, having been a skilled woodworker prior to becoming a monk, he went back to work to earn a living and take care of the child. He worked for a couple of years, making and repairing furniture for people from other villages, who appreciated his great skills.

The young girl, who was feeling terrible and couldn't hide her lies any longer, eventually told her parents the truth. They felt deeply ashamed and angry at their daughter. They hastily went to see the monk, apologized profusely, and asked to take the baby to live with them. They wanted to pay him back for the hardship. He replied, "Is that so?"

The monk said goodbye to the child and put his robes back on. He didn't want anything except to be a monk again and pray. He prayed for the parents, their daughter, their grandchild, and all the villagers, and they fed him until he passed away.

This, of course, is an unusual and exemplary state of equanimity, and possibly out of reach for most of us. It's more than likely that I would have complained about the blatant injustice of the unfounded accusations—an old trigger of mine. It requires a lot of discipline to exhibit transcendent behavior in an unjust situation. This story illustrates the workings of an extraordinary mind and an exquisite level of emotional intelligence. It inspires us to consider looking at things differently and, in some ways, model this kind of behavior: stop reacting, take a step back, reflect, and fare better as a result.

PRACTICING FORGIVENESS

Forgiveness means giving up all hope for a better past.

—Lily Tomlin

Post diagnosis, I took some time to regain perspective. Then I realized that I should ask for forgiveness from others I had hurt and forgive those who had caused harm to me. Cleaning the slate was a necessity for gaining peace of mind and feeling lighter. I invited the past to unfold in my mind and came up with a list of people who deserved an apology or two. I called, sent letters, and left messages on their phones.

When we have been betrayed, harmed, abandoned, and abused verbally or otherwise, we face an uphill path to forgiveness; it feels nothing short of impossible. Yet, keeping the anger or fear inside becomes unbearable. Resentment, a glacial attitude, or smoldering rage hardens us, deadens our spirits, and narrows our options for meeting what comes our way. Seeking revenge through anger gives us a false promise of relief, and everyone gets hurt in the process. Forgiveness releases us from the power of fear and retribution. It is not about superficiality, powerlessness, denying our hurt, or ignoring moments of cruelty and bitterness. We don't cover up our pain with a smile. Sometimes it takes time to be able to forgive and release our burdens. Eventually we muster up enough courage to forgive those who caused us harm, while remembering to use kind speech.

This is a difficult practice that requires humility, yielding, and surrender. "Humility" is derived from the Latin *humilis*, which means "returning to the ground," as if resting in the valley's richness because there is little that grows on mountaintops. When we open our hearts, we can see clearly that another's suffering has been projected onto us in a distorted fashion. We know this, because we too have been in similar states of mind at different junctures in our lives. When someone has harmed us, willingly or unwillingly, we can let go of the burden of plotting retaliation. It is not about the "other" anymore, it is all about freeing ourselves from unnecessary hardship.

BALANCE MEDITATION

We meditate to open what is closed, uncover what is hidden, calm what is reactive.

Be at ease in body, heart, and mind. Be at ease!

From the belly comes presence and intuition.

From the heart comes the wisdom of empathy and compassion.

From the head comes the wisdom of clarity and listening.

Rest in unobstructed awareness, letting go of the appearances of the mind.

Everything is movement, creation, and completion, like the waves of the sea coming and going, surging to shore and ebbing back to the vast ocean.

DEEPLY KNOWING WHAT MATTERS

The Well of Grief

Those who will not slip beneath
  the still surface on the well of grief,

turning down through its black water
  to the place we cannot breathe,

will never know the source from which we drink,
  the secret water, cold and clear,

nor find in the darkness glimmering,
  the small round coins,
    thrown by those who wished for something else.

(David Whyte 2006).

As I began to forgive myself and ask for forgiveness from others, I experienced a deeper knowing about the mystery of life. What really matters on the healing journey is whether we are content, and whether family and friends accept and love us for our basic humanity and goodness.

It is crucial, of course, that we meet our basic needs for safety, shelter, and food, before we approach meeting our higher emotional needs that shape us into decent and remarkable beings.

We don't need to identify with our mind states or emotions, and we certainly don't allow them to determine the nature of our experiences. One of our main errors, a delusion, is to believe that happiness derives essentially from outer circumstances, such as events or objects that will bring lasting feelings of satisfaction. When we realize this is false, we have the opportunity to make wholesome choices. Like the story of the monk who was accused of something he didn't do, we know deep within when we are aligned with our values and feel at ease, regardless of what others say or think.

Contentment is based on inner mental balance, which is an unwavering attitude of gently relating to circumstances that are neutral but often colored by our likes or dislikes, and other biases. By paying attention, we become aware of our afflictive thoughts and emotions and gain a deeper understanding of their source. This helps us discern whether they are constructive or not. If we can catch them early before they gain too much velocity, we will be better off.

Many Buddhist temples have all kinds of gaudy, menacing figures surrounding their entrances. They are a reminder that we leave our demons outside before we step into the sacred interior of our beings, where we meet ourselves over and over in our inner sanctums. Once there, we can be in awe of our strength, courage, tenacity, and will power. We can see each day as a blessed one.

Focusing on our intentions and not letting our minds be tugged back and forth by many distractions, we notice how powerful our intentions are, in and of themselves. They determine how we interpret and respond to information and provide a bridge between our values and goals. The more we understand the workings of our mind and consciousness, the better we are poised to contribute to our communities and influence our bodies' homeostasis, our mental health, and our spiritual well-being.

About a year after I was told I was cancer-free, I was inspired to provide others with the much-needed love and care I'd received myself. It took some time to figure out how I could serve others best. I went away and participated in a small three-day retreat to rest my mind, and the answer came to me clearly. My path was laid out to interact directly with people who have cancer and assist them on their journeys.

RC was a culinary professor, who loved everything about prepping and cooking food and feeding people. When he came to the group he had pancreatic recurrence, which is quite unusual. He had recently married a beautiful and kind woman. He knew this untimely second round of pancreatic cancer was going to be challenging and unpredictable. He hoped to stretch out living fully for as long as possible.

He kept teaching for a couple of years, until his energy waned. He left the support group, after attending once. "Not my cup of tea," he said, but joined the regular Sunday meditation group, favoring silence over talking. He gradually gained peace of mind and lived as if his life really mattered every minute. He consistently managed to arrive a couple of minutes before I rang the bell for the start of meditation.

I can still picture him, sitting in front of me on a zafuton. Even though he was experiencing physical discomfort, his face taking on darker shades of yellow and brown tints over the months, he never sat in a chair. But the life force was slowly, steadily, and forcibly disengaging. We often took a few minutes to check in or plan an individual session after the sit.

Then one Sunday, he didn't show up for himself. And then another. I kept sending him the dharma talks online, and we would occasionally converse on the phone, catching up about this and that. Then in early April, the last call came, with a request to visit him. When I arrived, his body was failing him. He was sitting on a couch, partially covered with a thick blanket, his skin leathery, his legs bloated like ill-fated balloons. The edema had heartlessly immobilized his limbs, allowing him to walk only a few feet at best.

RC was never tall, but now he looked smaller than I could have imagined. Across from him was the dining room, still covered with Christmas decorations in early spring. I didn't make any remarks as he said: "Christmas was nice, we were all together. A small pleasure. . . . You know, I am Italian, Catholic deep down. Now, I feel my loneliness in this sad, useless body. This is it, my friend. I hope to go on soon, as this is no way to be! I called you to thank you for the Sunday meditations I attended and for giving me the space to meet with you privately, when I needed personal support the most. Particularly when I was angry at being diagnosed again, while you were cancer-free. And I'd just found and married the woman I love most, only to lose her now. Could you lead one last meditation? The last one my dear friend. And it'd better be good!" He was too tired to smile, his eyes ablaze. I smiled for us both.

Fifteen minutes later he was nodding off. He woke up when I put my shoes on.

I got up, sat next to him, we hugged, no words were necessary. We had often touched our tenderness and feistiness together. Now we connected for the very the last time.

A few weeks later, a thousand people or more came to pay their respects and share memories about him. I officiated the memorial for his wife and immediate family members, while the streets around the funeral home became inundated with cars. People young and old waited outside to enter, not wanting to disturb the family members. He was a rock, who had provided nourishment and sustenance for many. RC had felt gratitude for serving so many people, and they extended their gratitude to his wife and family members in return, feeding their hearts, bringing them equanimity, and easing some grief in the process.

While teaching mindfulness classes, I often ask participants if they still have dinner together as a family. Sadly, not many do. This gives me an opportunity to strongly suggest they try to have a daily meal together and recount stories of rewarding moments that transpired during the day. This is not only an exercise in sharing wonderful surprises, but also a revelation of the positive experiences that feed and nourish everyone around the table. This abundance would otherwise be lost. When we appreciate the small gifts that consistently come our way, we feast from the horn of plenty.

MEDITATION ON THE FIVE ELEMENTS: A MEDITATION FOR HEALING

This meditation creates choices and facilitates restoring balance using the physical elements in nature to represent our bodies (earth), emotional stances (water), relationship styles (fire), states of mind (air), and spirituality (space). Depending on how much weight we habitually give each of them, sometimes too much or too little, each element has the capacity to exert wholesome or unwholesome effects in our lives.

EARTH ELEMENT

Wholesome aspects: Earth provides structure, security, stability, form, confidence, and an awareness of responsibility. It roots us in our experience and grounds us in pure being. We know this element well in nature: the trees we lean against, and the rocks we sit on. Notice what aspects of earth support you in life. Earth element is expressed in relationships by being supportive, protective, and nourishing. Mindfulness becomes easy when we are grounded, because the mind is stable, and insight naturally arises. In our spiritual practices, the earth element is the wisdom of equanimity fed by increasing knowledge.

Unwholesome aspects: When there is a lack of earth element, we lose touch with what is important, and we are easily knocked off balance. Too much earth element introduces qualities of dullness, inertia, literal thinking, apathy, insensitivity, and a lack of creativity. We invest in stability at any cost and become rigid or controlling in our immediate family circles and work settings.

WATER ELEMENT

Wholesome aspects: Water represents fluidity, navigating easily through life, finding comfort in oneself, accepting different conditions and situations, being content with people we meet and places we go. It inspires waves of joy, clarity, grief, and sadness. This element gives us a contentment in being alive that is innate, rather than dependent on external circumstances. When balanced, water helps us develop wisdom; our spiritual practice is to cultivate openness.

Unwholesome aspects: Too much water element produces complacency, oversensitivity, and a drifting mind that is lost in the ebb and flow of our emotions. We have little empathy, and we are too guarded, lacking understanding. We don't flow through our lives; instead, our feelings dam up and then leak. We channel them into narrow forms of expression. We get carried away.

FIRE ELEMENT

Wholesome aspects: Fire element's focus is on warmth, vitality, passion, intensity, intuition, enthusiasm, and joy in our creations and accomplishments. It brings excitement and wakes us up. Fire makes us feel passionate about people and things. We experience vividness and the wisdom of discernment. When out of balance, the spiritual practice is to increase generosity.

Unwholesome aspects: Excess fire makes us easily agitated, irritable, unstable, restless, and intolerant. It creates a lack of calm and peace. We might react impulsively and lack inspiration. Things and other people burn us up and consume us. There are things we can never get enough of. We don't finish projects. To reset, our spiritual practice is to overcome cravings and greed.

AIR ELEMENT

Wholesome aspects: Air is about movement, change, activity, and calm breath. It brings curiosity, flexibility of intellect, and the ability to change negative situations into positive ones. Air connects with everything and pervades everywhere. When challenged with too much air, the spiritual practice is to increase peace of mind.

Unwholesome aspects: When there is too much air element, we experience little stability or contentment, become fickle, and have difficulty accepting things as they are or finding comfort in them. We are unfocused, impatient, anxious, and in flight-mode. We don't explore new things or grow and expand with others. Practices related to air separate the pure and impure mind states.

SPACE ELEMENT

Wholesome aspects: Space represents boundlessness; everything arises, exists, and dissolves into space. It manifests as awareness. It enables us to accommodate whatever life brings, gives us tolerance, emotional capacities, and balance in most things. In relationships, it manifests as presence, giving us room to be who we are and allowing others to be themselves, without judgment. The wisdom of boundlessness is related to space, which has no defined limitations or specific center. When imbalanced, the spiritual practice is to increase love and compassion.

Unwholesome aspects: An overabundance of space shows up as not giving ourselves space for what we need to do, and for what or whom we care about. We can get spacey, which manifests as a feeling of losing touch, and experiencing a lack of awareness, presence, or meaning.

Most of us favor one or more of the five elements. This influences our physical constitution, emotional states, behavior, and mental traits. Through meditation we can explore both the wholesome and unwholesome aspects of each element to uncover our habitual tendencies. Then we can strengthen the ones that are deficient and lessen the ones that are dominant. When we achieve balance, we can live with difficult situations and few material possessions, remaining stable, centered, and flexible. When working with the five elements, we don't just use them as fillers or distractions in our lives; our connection with the elements is direct, the experience is vivid, and the possibilities for healing are unlimited.

While meditating on each of the five elements, symbols of great depth and long tradition, we move away from identifying with the content of our experience and toward living in the present moment, understanding that life is just a series of continuous moments we discern through many different lenses.

Conclusion

We all walk in shoes too small for us.

—Carl Jung

Some readers will be skeptical about my scientific assumptions and spiritual practices, or the mind-body relationship. In the past, I have attempted to find truth in science that didn't always answer the need for meaning in life. My study of Buddhism as a psychology and a way of life has shown me the value of human existence and offered unparalleled opportunities for realizing my higher potential. I have learned that to understand any discipline, one has to set an intention to practice it.

Jung's words suggest that we need to choose new ideas, preferrable mind states, and noble aspirations with which to face the challenges and blessings of life, health, and illness, without limiting new, viable approaches to change that will let us flourish. We have to believe that we are capable of walking the path best suited for us, allowing nothing to stop us from exploring our outer and inner worlds, one step and one revelation at a time.

The cancer odyssey feels overwhelming when we don't know what the future will offer. We must alter our attitude on several occasions and rely on effort, discipline, intuition, insight, kindness, and faith. Using the acronym ATTITUDE to explore what we experience and discern the available choices that will move us toward well-being brings into focus everything that is needed to go beyond battling cancer. Many of the meditation practices and exercises within each chapter are perspectives and insights gained over forty-five years from revered teachers and traditions. These practices bring meaning and guidance during illness, but they also provide a pragmatic analysis of the reality of suffering and how we might become free of it.

A meditation practice involves open-minded inquiry that informs our view of the world. It gradually alters our outlook and results in changes in our conduct and way of life. This influences our values and leads to important shifts and self-transformation. Insights into the nature of the mind gained through the practice of meditation are designed to heal mental afflictions. Introspection enables us to identify which mental processes are beneficial and which are harmful and make choices based on this knowledge. Navigating uncertainty during the journey demands that we deconstruct roadblocks of old, habitual patterns. Changing our relation to our thoughts encourages the active cultivation of qualities such as courage, patience, love, temperance, learned optimism, and faith in something greater than ourselves. Our minds are not intrinsically imbalanced, even during illness. With skilled effort, a state of well-being that is not just contingent upon sensory, intellectual, behavioral, or aesthetic stimuli will grow and mature.

I have witnessed many cancer patients become free of rogue cells, or live much longer than predicted—five, ten, twenty years—and suffer less, because they changed their attitudes. There is also specific, concrete, scientific evidence to support my observations. Research has shown that patients diagnosed with breast, lung, colon, and other cancers who practiced mindfulness and made lifestyle changes similar to those described in this book, experienced a reduction in levels of depression, anxiety, fatigue, and sleep deprivation, and their quality of life improved.

More research is called for to validate markers of change due to the cultivation of practices resulting from a kind attitude toward oneself. Epigenetics, neuroscience, and studies of the mind and consciousness continue to show that cultivating kindness and compassion, combined with allopathic medical interventions, is more effective than the restrictive and paltry goal of survivorship. Many recovered patients, cancer-free after months or years of treatments, will readily announce that we are grateful for the journey. We've risen from the ashes like a phoenix with a fresh understanding of the meaning and purpose of life. Instead of hanging by our teeth from a branch, high above solid ground, we speak our minds with words of gratitude and humility, savoring the meaning behind the words. We don't have a need to convince anyone else or beg that they change their views. We stand tall again, as living examples of the many possibilities for moving beyond illness to experience freedom from suffering.

LAST MEDITATION

Envision yourself sitting in your favorite chair, perhaps a rocking chair on a lovely porch, looking at the horizon that extends far away. There is nothing preventing you from seeing the fine line where the ground and sky dissolve.

You are very comfortable and watch the sun drop behind that line. You contemplate and reminisce about the past ninety years of your life.

Who knew what life was offering you? Who knew how it was going to unfold? Who knew what you brought to it, often with conviction?

Here you are now, fully contemplating the answers to the following questions:

- What happy memories will I share with family and friends?
- What have been the most rewarding and meaningful moments in this amazing life of mine?
- What lessons and insights have I gained that made me this very decent human being?
- Does anyone come to mind who I need to forgive or ask for forgiveness from?
- Whom and what am I grateful for in this long life?
- What lingering regrets do I have, and will I be able to let them go?
- What wishes do I have for all the people that I am close to?

Now, come back to the present moment and explore how these thoughts and insights might inform your life now.

Once you have clarity, let go, contemplate the horizon right where earth and sky meet in oneness.

Postscript

Even after all this time, the sun never says to the earth, you owe me. Look what happens with a love like that! It lights up the whole sky!

—Hafiz

I knew, from working in healthcare systems for decades, that the odds of recovery from a stage IV cancer diagnosis were slim. Unable to sleep or eat much, I was weak, foggy, and absentminded. I had ample time on my hands, yet I couldn't muster enough energy to use it. Several times, I had to summon a shift in attitude so I could lift myself up by my bootstraps. I often felt that words were either overwrought or inadequate to describe the fears, trepidation, and anger surrounding my declining élan vital.

The pivotal ATTITUDE outlined here supported me in my diagnosis, treatment, and recovery. I can now view my experience and struggles with balance and perspective. However, it wasn't always easy to motivate myself to change mind states. On a few occasions, I wallowed in pity, as physical limitations caused an overwhelming sense of futility to surface. When I felt ill at ease in my changed body, I needed courage to stand side by side with others and connect. Loneliness, as an alternative, was too devastating.

When chemotherapy treatment ended, I became gradually healthier and would take short walks. There was a cemetery not too far from where I lived, with a number of graves dating from the time of the early settlers up to the end of the First World War. The German word for cemetery, *Friedhof*, means "field of peace." It was a restorative place for me, where each evening squirrels, birds, chipmunks, and deer spent the last hours of the day.

I pondered the lives of those buried there, from the days before cars, electronics, and all the conveniences we take for granted. Most of the dead had common names; a surprising number died in infancy; a handful lived into their seventies; a large number were women. I wondered if they were remembered, and if so, what they were remembered for.

I lay there on the moss carpet, among the graves, enjoying the quiet and gazing every now and then at the lively animals, who didn't mind my presence. The evening sun was gradually descending beyond the slate headstones, most of them damaged by years of harsh New England winters. Fireflies would eventually light up the area, flashing intermittently. Some folklore has it that they are the remains of fallen stars flickering in the dark. I contemplated the profundity of my precious and fragile life, among the spirits of those who had departed to another realm. I was grateful then and I'm grateful now.

Cure has its limitations. The mind, on the other hand, is unbounded and a powerful tool with which to focus on quality-of-life options. With an open mind, there are multiple opportunities to experience well-being. The yearning to heal manifests when we choose to go to the tender, emotional places where we were absent before. Dealing with a cancer diagnosis is not a matter of tolerating the cards we are dealt or resigning ourselves to a tough-luck capitulation. We each have the capacity to modify our responses, the potential to project our imaginations beyond an assumed fait accompli, and the opportunity to adopt new vistas of human life.

On my journey, I asked for what I needed and received many gifts of insight and tenderness. These often melted away my disappointments, although the grieving process was real. The many ways we show up for ourselves, over and over, particularly in areas of uncharted territory, is nothing short of remarkable. The more we stay in the moment with wakefulness, instead of wishing for something else, the more we become aware of significant possibilities and readily dismiss fear-based probabilities. Amazing and wonderful people show up with support, food, time, prayers, and good wishes. Some are acquaintances, many are strangers; all tend to our needs as best they know how to, even as we wish to be invisible, feeling naked and so vulnerable.

No matter what the outcome would be for me biologically speaking, and regardless of the length of my temporal existence, I was firmly invested in improving my quality of life. Whether recovering or dying, we can still be fully alive while relying on the breath. It takes strength to accept the different chapters of the ever-changing life continuum and turn the pages without knowing what the tome might hold in store. I was determined not to close the book, or skip any of the chapters due to regret, rancor, destructive emotions, or unfulfilled wishes. I didn't want my heart to be filled with relentless anger, disappointments, or resentment. I aimed to live fully and find new meaning, purpose, and a new vocation post-disease.

I didn't want to be the same person I was prior to being ill. My identity was too closely related to professional life, taking care of business, accomplishing lots of tasks, and functioning on autopilot mode. When I reflected on mortality, I realized what was most important: longing to belong and espousing values that shaped me into a decent and kind human being. I reflected on what surprised and inspired me, and how much I'd learned about love.

Cultivating compassion for ourselves, ATTITUDE gives us courage for deep inquiry into the workings of the body, heart, and mind and helps us chart clear coordinates to thrive—not just endure—with determination. It helps us cultivate self-compassion and tenderly manage life's unexpected and paradoxical situations. When we are on a sacred journey, it is impossible to hold on to the past. Accepting the present is how we discover unknown dimensions of being and welcome the universal breath of life. The mystery of the journey with all its many detours and turns will ultimately be revealed.

People often ask me, as a chaplain, how I bear the immense and continuous suffering, the witnessing of so many deaths? It is a fair question and there are a couple of ways I respond. One answer I give is that I took vows, called the Four Great Bodhisattva Vows. This is a code of ethics that Buddhist students might pledge to adhere to under the guidance of a root teacher, to become invested in relieving the suffering of fellow beings through compassionate acts. The oath is always sacred and voluntary, rather than commanded. It is a set of aspirations we endeavor to live up to:

The Four Great Bodhisattva Vows

- Creations are numberless, I vow to free them.
- Delusions are inexhaustible, I vow to transform them.
- Reality is boundless, I vow to perceive it.
- The awakened way is unsurpassable, I vow to embody it.

My second reply is that I benefit greatly from observing the multiple ways people face stress, illness, and loss, and how they come to terms with and integrate them. I am surprised to see what illuminates their paths and what they are passionate about. I can never guess by looking at someone how they meet and direct the life force within, nor do I need to judge them. Observing how they deal with impermanence and unwanted surprises, and how they discover the depth of their resolve and vulnerability, speaks volumes to me. I don't internalize their suffering; I practice self-care and self-compassion. There is little room in the support groups for banalities and idle chatter, yet laughter and tears abound. Most cancer patients adopt new learning, welcome exploration, and honor connectivity.

Chaplains adhere to many precepts, such as not killing the mind of compassion, honoring life, and not taking what doesn't belong. I have combined them all into one abiding principle: create no separation.

To all I have been privileged to meet, and all those I will meet one day, I bow humbly. I honor each one, supporting them in exploring their vast interior life and the wisdom that proceeds from it. I am grateful to meet so many courageous and inspiring beings and witness their innate kindness for each other. I often greet them when they are most vulnerable, after their initial diagnosis, and share companionship with them as they embark on their unexpected adventure. Yet their journey is especially designed for them, contains everything needed for them to grow, and reveals glimpses of what needs to be explored in a different light. Being amid those who suffer and bearing witness to their zest for vividness makes my heart flame with luminosity.

And those who shed their bodies along the way keep mingling their spirits and memories among us to reveal what is essential: kindness, bravery, connection, belonging, and decency. The sun's light shifts during the seasons, but it continues to shine.

Let it be so!

References

1. American Cancer Society. 2019. "Cancer mortality milestone: 25 years of continuous decline." Accessed July 6, 2020. http://pressroom.cancer.org/Statistics2019.

2. Centers for Disease Control and Prevention. n.d. "Expected new cancer cases and deaths in 2020." https://www.cdc.gov/cancer/dcpc/research/articles/cancer_2020.htm. Accessed July 6, 2020.

3. Chödrön, Pema. 2019, December 06. "How We Get Hooked by Shenpa." *Lion's Roar.* https://www.lionsroar.com/how-we-get-hooked-shenpa-and-how-we-get-unhooked/.

4. Church, Dawson. 2014. *The genie in your genes: Epigenetic Medicine and the New Biology of Intention.* Santa Rosa, CA: Energy Psychology Press.

5. Coyle, Virginia, and Jack Zimmerman. 1996. *The way of council.* Bramble Books.

6. Davidson, Richard J., and Sharon Begley. 2012. *The Emotional Life of Your Brain: How Its Unique Patterns Affect the Way You Think, Feel, and Live--and How You Can Change Them,* 3rd ed. New York: Hudson Street Press.

7. Dorval, Marcelle. *Le Coeur sur la Main.* 1943. New York: Brentano's.

8. Goleman, Daniel, and Richard. J. Davidson. 2017. *Altered traits. Science Reveals How Meditation Changes Your Mind, Brain, and Body.* New York: Avery.

9. Goleman, Daniel. (2003). *Healing emotions: Conversations with the Dalai Lama on Mindfulness, Emotions, and Health.* Boulder, CO: Shambhala.

10. Goleman, Daniel. 1998. *Working with emotional intelligence.* New York: Bantam Books.

11. Kabat-Zinn, Jon. (2012). *Mindfulness for beginners: Reclaiming the present moment—and your life.* Colorado: Sounds True, Inc.

12. Kolata, Gina. 2013. "Hopeful glimmers in long war on cancer." *The New York Times,* November 4, 2013. https://www.nytimes.com/2013/11/04/booming/hopeful-glimmers-in-long-war-on-cancer.html.

13. Lipton, Bruce. 2008. *The Biology of Belief: Unleashing the Power of Consciousness, Matter, & Miracles.* California: Hay House.

14. Mountain Dreamer, Oriah. 1999. *The Invitation.* San Francisco: HarperONE.

15. National Cancer Institute. 2018, April 27. "Cancer statistics."

16. https://www.cancer.gov/about-cancer/understanding/statistics.

17. Nolan, K. 2002. "Death expert is facing her own." *Arizona Republic*, October 19. Phoenix, AZ.

18. O'Donohue, J. 2008. *To bless the space between us.* New York: Doubleday.

19. Remen, Rachel Naomi. 2000. *My grandfather's blessings: Stories of strength, refuge and belonging.* New York: Riverhead Books.

20. Rilke, Rainer Maria. 2013. *Letters to a Young Poet.* New York: Penguin Books.

21. Rinpoche, Anyen, and Allison Choying Zangmo. 2013. *The Tibetan Yoga of Breath: Breathing Practices for Healing the Body and Cultivating Wisdom.* Shambala.

22. Siegel, D. J. 2017. *Mind: A journey to the heart of being human.* New York: W.W. Norton & Co.

23. Siegel, D. 2021. "Mindsight." https://drdansiegel.com/mindsight/.

24. Wallace, B. Alan. 2009. *Mind in the balance: Meditation in science, Buddhism, and Christianity.* New York: Columbia University Press.

25. Watson, G., Batchelor, S., and Claxton, C. eds. 2012. *The psychology of awakening.* York Beach, Maine: Samuel Weiser.

26. Whyte, David. 2006. *River Flow: New and Selected Poems.* Langley, Washington: Many Rivers Press.

27. Whyte, David. 1997. *The House of Belonging.* Langley, Washington: Many Rivers Press.

Endorsements

"A beautiful book, written from the heart. True, rich and actionable. I highly recommend this remarkable exploration of cancer with an attitude."

Roshi Joan Halifax, PhD

Abbot, Upaya Zen Center, Santa Fe

" I find the book beautifully and insightfully written in a way that will be of great benefit for people with cancer at all stages of their journey, including physicians and caregivers. The wisdom in the text informed by your own experience mingled with interesting anecdotes is a book that will be well received.

I seek your permission to share it with patients who will benefit from it."

Michael Castro, MD

Board certified in Neuro-Oncology and Medical Oncology

"Pierre Zimmerman provides us with the insights of both a patient and a healer in facing the suffering of cancer.

Medical students and resident physicians will benefit from the book's lessons: that those with serious illness can be helped to achieve peace of mind and be fully alive, no matter how long, or how brief, the journey."

Gerald Klaus Schynoll, MD,MPH, FACP Associate Professor of Medicine, Albany Medical College

"Beyond Survivorship is a must for those diagnosed with cancer, those that love them, and those that help them. This book is not a memoir, but rather a moving and compelling plan of action and practices that offer resiliency, hope and transformation to guide beings and thrive beyond their diagnosis."

Ann Saffi Biasetti, PhD, LCSWR

Author of Befriending Your Body: A Self Compassionate Approach to Freeing Yourself From Disordered Eating and Awakening Self Compassion Cards.

"Your book is absolutely spectacular and should be required reading in every Medical School and Nursing Curriculum. I am eager to have it made available to recommend to my patients, friends and colleagues. This is a great gift of knowledge that you give to the world and I see the cancer as only a side line in this story that will benefit all that read it. It will have a huge impact on the lives of everyone that has the good fortune to read it. For me, personally, it has been transformative."

Joseph W Bell, MD, FACS

Castle ConnollyTop Surgeon

When I got my cancer diagnosis, I could certainly have used this book. Luckily, I joined one of the support groups, Pierre led. I see wisdom in the pages of 'Cancer with An Attitude'. It is important to realize that even in illness we have choices. Pierre shows that with an attitude we can diminish the destructive power of harmful emotions and harness energy towards constructive thinking that supports healing.

The book doesn't disparage conventional medical treatment and applies timeless wisdom practices for the person with cancer and their loved ones. "Making the most of this precious life" is what we all hope for.

Ellen

I was glad as a twenty year old to be exposed to life skills that I would more than likely never have learned, being so young, without having been diagnosed with cancer!

The opportunity to be with people of all ages, female and male, sharing similar challenging journeys in the support group was an eye opener. It gave me the ability to look at life in a way I would have never benefited otherwise, since most of my friends had a difficult time showing up for me, not interested in hanging around, instead experimenting with drugs, one even died from an overdose.

I am grateful, every day, for waking up to what is important in my life now that I am cancer free. I am dating a nice person, something new for me. The awareness, the deep connections I gained, and living with a positive outlook are the best gifts I cherish. I think this book is going to be meaningful for many people who have cancer.

Josie

This book is precious, because it gave me the chance to have an attitude that brought relief in the midst of darkness and confusion. I am fortunate I was involved with the support groups and mindfulness classes available. They opened my eyes to what is important: the opportunity to make the most of my life now that I am cancer free. Being with others who were diagnosed with cancer, invested in growing, in spite of not knowing what the future holds, gave me renewed purpose and the willingness to become a much more decent human being than I was, prior to my diagnosis. I am truly blessed!

Harry